Cesarean Section

A Johns Hopkins Press Health Book

Michele Moore
M.D., FAAFP

Caroline de Costa
M.D., FRCOG, FRANZCOG, MPH

ﾞ ﾞ ﾞ

Cesarean Section
Understanding and Celebrating Your Baby's Birth

The Johns Hopkins University Press
BALTIMORE AND LONDON

Note to the Reader. This book embodies our approach to gynecological and obstetric practice and to Cesarean section in general. It was not written about *your* pregnancy or your situation. Although we believe and practice its philosophy, we adjust our approach to suit each patient's particular need and each family's situation. Obviously, we would not treat you without first learning a great deal about you, and so your treatment should not be based solely on what is written here. It must be developed in a dialogue between you and your physician. Our book is written to help you with that dialogue.

Drawings by Jacqueline Schaffer; photographs by Dr. Paul Howat.

© 2003 The Johns Hopkins University Press
All rights reserved. Published 2003
Printed in the United States of America on acid-free paper
9 8 7 6 5 4 3 2 1

The Johns Hopkins University Press
2715 North Charles Street
Baltimore, Maryland 21218-4363
www.press.jhu.edu

Library of Congress Cataloging-in-Publication Data

Moore, Michele
   Cesarean section : understanding and celebrating your baby's birth / Michele Moore, Caroline de Costa.
        p. cm.
Includes bibliographical references and index.
   ISBN 0-8018-7336-3 (hdbk. : alk. paper) — ISBN 0-8018-7337-1 (pbk.)
   1. Cesarean section—Popular works.   I. De Costa, Caroline, 1947– II. Title.
RG761 .M664   2003
618.4—dc21   2002013625
6 18.86
A catalog record for this book is available from the British Library.

Contents

APPENDIXES

Acknowledgments

Many people have been supportive and helpful in the course of this project.

Thank you to the women who gave us your stories—you know who you are.

Thank you to Jean Slepian, librarian extraordinaire, who procured many journal articles for us. Also, thanks to the library staff of Cairns Base Hospital.

Thank you to our editor, Jacqueline Wehmueller, who was there for us.

Thank you to Dr. Paul Howat, who took the very sensitive photographs of a Cesarean birth. Also thank you to the young family—Clinton, Jody, and Damon—who agreed to share this intimate time with us.

We could not have written this book without the support and patience of our families and staffs. Michele wants especially to thank Martin and Anneke for the experience of being their Cesarean Mom. It has been a great gift. Caroline feels much gratitude to her children Javed, Sophie, and Naomi and thanks Josie Valese for help with the vagaries of computers.

Cesarean Section

Introduction

Two months ago, Jan and Paul began sharing in the joy of caring for their lovely baby boy, named Daniel Matthew after both grandfathers. Jan has four months of maternity leave left before she will return to work part time. Paul works from home and will be able to take care of Daniel. To top off all the goodies, Daniel is breast-feeding very well and—incredible luck—already sleeps through the night.

So why is Jan sitting in Michele's office, crying her eyes out? This office visit was supposed to be for a routine checkup and to show off the baby to Jan's family physician. "It was all so different from what we had planned and dreamed about," Jan explains tearfully, "different from our birth plan and from what we learned in childbirth class. I expected to be in control! I didn't expect so much pain! I thought I'd have an easy delivery! I never expected that my cervix would refuse to dilate or that Daniel's heartbeat would slow down. It was so scary, and then, to have a C-section! I never, ever considered that I might have a C-section."

Jan had had an uneventful pregnancy. She ate healthy foods, took her prenatal vitamins, walked daily, swam, exercised gently at the gym, and was careful to sleep eight hours every night. She gave up coffee (it made her sick to her stomach) and the glass of wine she and Paul had usually enjoyed with dinner. Jan and Paul had shared the daily erotic experience of his massaging her perineum (the area between the vagina and the rectum) with vitamin E oil to help make the skin flexible enough to slip easily over the baby's head during delivery.

This was going to be a perfect birth, they had decided, and they both wanted it to be a perfect experience, too. They read childbirth books together and watched videotapes of childbirth. They played Chopin and bagpipe music to in utero Zhivago (their before-birth name for their baby) with the idea that one would soothe his soul and the other would get him pumping his muscles. Paul loved spooning in bed with Jan and feeling Zhivago's gentle kicks in his back.

Both Jan and Paul attended every one of the childbirth classes at the hospital and drew up the following birth plan:

1. Jan won't be induced unless there is a good medical reason.
2. To help control discomfort, Jan and Paul will use heat, water, massage, and breathing exercises.
3. Paul will be present at all times.
4. No epidural or other drugs.
5. No episiotomy.

The due date came . . . and went! Everything remained fine: Jan's blood pressure and weight, the baby's heart rate and movements. Ten days passed.

On day 11, Jan awoke to the warm, wet sensation of her membranes rupturing. At first she thought she had wet the bed, but then she felt faint cramps and realized her water had broken. She woke Paul, they called the obstetrician, and five minutes later they were on their way to the hospital.

After checking in through the Emergency Room, Jan was wheeled up to her room in the obstetric suite. She was encouraged to walk around the room and in the corridor. She walked . . . and walked . . . and walked. Nothing happened except the odd twinge. All day she walked, and then she slept fitfully through the night. Paul was draped over a lounge chair, bleary-eyed. Both Jan and Paul were frustrated at the lack of action. What had happened to their perfect experience?

Come morning, the obstetrician advised starting a Pitocin drip to induce contractions. Disappointed, Jan and Paul reluctantly agreed. Now Jan was walking around with a tall, skinny friend—her IV pole. She spent some time watching television in her room with Paul. Periodically the nurse checked her progress. Four hours after the "pit" was started, Jan's cervix was dilated only two centimeters. Still eight centimeters to go! But it was progress.

With a feeling of accomplishment, Jan walked the halls some more. Soon, though, a nagging suspicion began to niggle at her that there was more than "discomfort" in this childbirth business. She soaked in a soothing warm-water bath and Paul massaged her back, but the pain was getting worse!

A few minutes later, Jan was back in bed asking the nurse for some pain medication. An injection of Demerol made things better for a while, but soon she felt as if she was being torn in two. Covered in sweat, she twisted and turned in the bed. And then, to her great embarrassment, she heard herself screaming. Paul stood by, terrified. He begged Jan to try the epidural, to help her save her strength for delivering Zhivago. Now, telling Michele this story, Jan is again feeling embarrassed. How could she have been so out of control?

It seemed to take forever for the anesthesiologist to arrive. Jan was hoping she would just pass out and escape the pain, she tells Michele. Finally, the epidural was in place. Jan says: "I felt a blessed numbness in my belly. I could feel the contractions with my hands on my belly, but the pain of the contractions was gone. The nurse gave me a button to push to control how much drug went in through the epidural, and I actually slept until the change of shift."

Over the next six hours, Jan's belly contracted rhythmically, but her cervix was only five centimeters dilated. The fetal monitor then showed that the baby was distressed, and a blood sample taken from his scalp confirmed this. The obstetrician explained to Paul and Jan that it would be many more hours before Jan's cervix would be dilated enough for a vaginal delivery. The safest thing for the baby would be an immediate Cesarean section. Now frightened, Jan and Paul agreed.

I was so sad as I left the birthing room, all peach and chintz, and was rolled down the hall on a stretcher. We even had soft music in the birthing suite, and now that was gone, too. They rolled me into an icy-cold, white room and put blue paper things on me: a robe, slippers, and a shower cap. When I looked, Paul was covered in blue, too. They told him to sit down in a corner. And I *needed* him. Everybody else was busy with their jobs, and Paul couldn't even hold my hand. Then, before I could ask any questions, they set up a paper-covered frame between my face and my belly. I could hear instruments being moved around on a table. I couldn't feel my belly and I couldn't see it. It was like my belly and our baby existed only in my imagination.

Next, I felt a strange sensation: first pressure and then a queer empty feeling that made me woozy. The anesthesiologist put something in my IV, and the faint feeling passed. And then, I heard a cry! It was Daniel. The obstetrician was holding him up, and he was so slippery looking, with dark-green slimy stuff all over his legs. The pediatrician whisked Daniel away, and I don't remember much more. Paul says he went with the pediatrician to the nursery while I was sewn up, and I didn't really wake up until about five hours later. I know I was exhausted.

I feel like I failed the most important test in my life. I couldn't even give birth to my own baby. *And* I screamed and humiliated myself.

The next day, Jan told Michele, her feelings of failure had not improved. Myra and Natalie, her friends from childbirth classes, were also in the obstetric suite, and both of them had "done it"! Only forty minutes after arriving at the hospital, Myra had delivered her baby, Paige. Natalie had had a little more trouble and had an epidural, but her baby, Stefan, also arrived just fine. Both admitted that the whole experience was more painful than they had ever imagined, but that was little comfort to Jan.

Then Greta, the childbirth educator, had breezed in and heartily congratulated Myra and Natalie before spending half an hour telling Jan how sorry she was, better luck next time—confirming Jan's feeling that she hadn't done it right.

"Ever since I went home, I've been going over and over it all, trying to figure out what I did wrong. It must be my fault," Jan told Michele.

Michele could imagine how it had been at home: Jan with a healing incision on her belly, a bladder with little control, and a bowel performing sluggishly. Being able to move around more easily might have helped Jan work out some of her feelings, but she had been forced to take it easy and so she had brooded on her "failure." Fortunately, Daniel is an easy baby.

Jan's examination that afternoon was postponed to another day, and Michele spent the visit explaining to Jan that C-section is never anybody's "fault." Sometimes nature just doesn't get labor and childbirth right. In the past, unfortunately, when things did not go right, many women and babies died during childbirth. So ask yourself, Is the point of childbirth delivering a baby the way nature intended or having a healthy baby and mother?

"When you put it that way," Jan agreed, "it's pretty clear we had a good outcome, because Daniel is healthy. But I still can't help feeling disappointed, because it wasn't anything like what we had expected or planned for."

Going into labor for the first time always involves entering unknown territory because your body has never done this before. First-time labor tends to be longer, less efficient, and riskier, especially for the baby. About 70 percent of first-time labors end with a vaginal delivery of a healthy baby; 30 percent do not.

What happens in the 30 percent of first-time labors and deliveries that don't go smoothly? Some labors start fine but then slow down and stop, even when Pitocin is used to help stimulate contractions. Sometimes the baby becomes distressed, as Daniel did. Some of these distressed babies would die or be permanently injured if the labor was allowed to continue to vaginal delivery. Sometimes the mother's health problems (such as diabetes, high blood pressure, or hemorrhage) endanger the life of the baby or the mother even before labor starts. Then the baby may have to be delivered immediately, sometimes by Cesarean section, and possibly before the baby's due date. Some women would never be able to deliver their babies vaginally, and the lives of both mother and baby would be endangered without a Cesarean delivery. Some babies are delivered vaginally with the assistance of forceps.

In the 30 percent of difficult births, Cesarean section has become the safest medical option for a safe delivery—safer in most cases than a forceps delivery. Forceps, once widely used, carry a greater risk of birth injuries to mother and baby than does C-section. In most developed countries and for some fortunate women in less developed regions, Cesarean section is today a widely available option for difficult births. The C-section rate in developed countries is 20–25 percent of all births. Medical procedures that are performed frequently and are widely available are safer because doctors routinely practice performing such procedures and have available a vast cumulative experience. C-section in many cases saves lives—and yet, Jan and Paul's childbirth books devoted only a few pages to it, mostly providing advice about how to avoid a Cesarean birth. And their birthing classes had not prepared them for a Cesarean birth, either.

No one knows the "correct" rate of Cesarean birth, and there are ongoing arguments over the rate being too high or too low (see chap. 1). In developed countries, however, the rate hovers around 20–25 percent, regardless of differences in health insurance coverage and health care philosophy. In the United States, the United Kingdom, Ireland, and Western Europe, the rate of C-section is around 22 percent of all births.

In our view, because up to a quarter of all births are Cesarean births, *prenatal preparation should include information about Cesarean section for every woman.* And that is why we have written this guide. We will look at why C-sections are sometimes necessary and at what happens during the procedure and afterward. This realistic guide is for prospective parents, for whom C-section is a possibility that must be considered, as well as for parents who have given birth to a child by C-section and who may still be disappointed or confused or feel that they failed. We will explore why Jan's feelings of disappointment are so common among modern-day mothers. The information in this book will also be helpful for women who have had C-sections but do not experience such feelings.

In the 1970s a backlash against the increasing "medicalization" of birth brought demands for "natural childbirth" (that is, birth without anesthesia, forceps, or other medical intervention) and fostered parents' mistrust of medical care providers involved in birth. Birth became political and was increasingly seen as an extension of women's rights over their bodies. A chasm exists still between midwives and obstetricians, and the lack of dialogue between them is one reason C-section is often seen as a second-best option, to be avoided if at all possible.

"Once a C-section, always a C-section" is no longer a truism. A woman who has previously delivered by Cesarean section can deliver vaginally next time, if her health and other conditions allow. But in our view the movement to avoid repeat Cesarean sections has been carried too far, and some women feel that they cannot choose a planned and well-controlled repeat C-section because it is not socially acceptable. Some women want the option of having a Cesarean birth on demand and meet with strong opposition from their doctor, their family and friends, and their health insurance plan.

To help explain the controversy over C-section, we will describe the history of the surgery as well as the more recent political squabbles. We'll give you lots of information about the surgery itself: why it may be necessary, what the experience is like, and how to cope afterward. We'll talk about risks and complications of the procedure and prospects for future births, and we'll help you develop questions to ask your own doctor or midwife.

Our perspective is that a *Cesarean section is simply another way to give birth.* The most satisfying, empowering, and rewarding part of birth is not pushing a baby through your vagina, but holding your healthy infant in your arms and knowing that you are responsible for his or her life.

We know about pregnancy, birth, and C-sections. We are both mothers, and we both take care of women. Caroline, the mother of seven children, became a specialist obstetrician/gynecologist and has performed several thousand Cesarean sections. She obviously has extensive experience with the joys as well as the pitfalls of pregnancy and childbirth. Her children were all delivered vaginally, but soon after her last baby, she had a hysterectomy and surgery for pelvic floor repair. So she also knows what gynecological surgery is like from personal experience.

Michele became a family physician who went on to practice preventive care, mostly women's health, and to become an expert on menopause. Michele's two children were born by C-section, one emergency and one scheduled repeat. Between us, we have more than 50 years' experience of caring for women. We wrote this book to share our experience and our accumulated wisdom with you.

We believe strongly that it is time to speak out and say that Cesarean section is a *normal* birth method and that women who have a Cesarean section should not be made to feel that they have failed. When things do not go as planned, some disappointment is natural, but we want to help mothers (and fathers, too) get past the disappointment. It's worth repeating that the goal in childbirth is to ensure the arrival of a healthy baby whom you will mother, with all that implies, for the rest of your life. What counts is the bonding of this special loving relationship.

We hope you find the information in this book useful and helpful in thinking about C-section, whether you have already had a Cesarean and want to understand the experience better, you wish to plan for another C-section birth, or you are expecting a baby and want to be informed about all the possibilities ahead, including this other normal way of bringing a baby into the world.

PART I

ࣔ ࣔ ࣔ

THE WHY, WHAT, AND WHEN
OF CESAREAN SECTION

CHAPTER 1

ॐ ॐ ॐ

Why Are Cesarean Sections Performed?

As the stories in this book illustrate, there are many reasons for having a Cesarean section, ranging from dire emergency to planned choice. But there are many people who don't have access to accurate information about Cesarean section, and their ideas about C-section come from the media. Media discussions about Cesarean deliveries tend not to tell the whole story, however, and generally do not focus on the lives saved because of Cesarean delivery. Instead, the media focus on the percentages of Cesarean births (the current rate is 22–25% in developed countries).

Let us start this chapter, then, by remedying this situation. People need to know that *Cesarean births represent births that, before modern obstetric practice, often resulted in tragedy.* Today, it is rare for a mother or baby to die from the birth process. Modern techniques for surgical birth save lives: Cesarean section is a modern remedy.

Before proceeding, we must define exactly what is meant by elective or planned and by emergency or nonelective C-sections. These definitions are so important that they are repeated in the glossary.

An *emergency C-section* is just that: it is urgent and is done to save the life of the mother or baby, either or both of whom are in immediate danger. It is performed for unexpected medical reasons that occur during pregnancy or labor. The term *nonelective C-section* is used interchangeably with the term *emergency C-section*.

An *elective C-section* is *not* an unnecessary C-section or a

C-section done for the convenience of the mother or doctor. An elective C-section is done for medical reasons that are known ahead of time (for example, the mother may have a large fibroid blocking the birth canal). Because the mother's medical situation is known before labor begins, the surgery can be planned for a specific time near the baby's due date. The term *planned C-section* is used interchangeably with the term *elective C-section*.

Obviously, there are times when the margins get blurred. A planned C-section can become more urgent if labor starts. Or a known medical condition may worsen during pregnancy, making an emergency C-section necessary. The major point is that *all of these C-sections are done for good medical reasons*.

In recent years, some women have expressed the wish to have their babies by C-section even though there is no compelling medical reason for a Cesarean delivery. This kind of C-section, called *C-section on demand* or *C-section on request*, is exceedingly rare in the United States or Australia, but it is common in South America and increasingly so in Great Britain. The argument for C-section on demand is that it preserves the woman's pelvic floor and prevents future problems and surgeries for incontinence and prolapse. This book is not about this option.

We think that decisions about delivery should be made by the pregnant woman herself whenever possible and that women should have access to all the information they need to make the best decisions for themselves and their families. The decisions should be based on up-to-date and complete medical information, on the kind and level of expertise available where the woman will give birth, and on the specific needs of the mother and baby and the rest of the family. When it comes to delivering a baby, complete information includes the information that, *sometimes, decisions must be made urgently*. Every pregnant woman will be better prepared if she understands that a Cesarean section is sometimes necessary and that, in these circumstances, there really is no other good choice.

The Reasons for Cesarean Deliveries Today

Today, 30 percent of Cesareans are repeat C-sections. Usually, the reason for this is transparent: the condition that made Cesarean delivery necessary previously still exists in this pregnancy. Until the past couple of decades, a woman who had had a Cesarean delivery for any reason would automatically be scheduled for a repeat C-section for any subsequent pregnancy. If she unexpectedly went into labor, a C-section was immediately performed. Today, in some circumstances, a woman may opt for a trial of labor for a vaginal birth after a previous C-section. Vaginal birth after C-section is discussed in chapter 10.

Failure to progress in labor accounts for another 30 percent of Cesareans. Failure to progress is due to a combination of factors: the size and flexibility of the mother's pelvis, the strength of contractions, and the position of the baby. *Cephalopelvic disproportion* is the term used to describe the situation when the mother's pelvis won't allow the baby to move along the birth canal. In this situation the woman *can't* give birth vaginally, any more than she could stretch her mouth around a whole watermelon. The baby may be particularly big, or the mother's pelvis may be naturally small, or there may simply be a disproportion between the two. The force of the contractions is another factor. Both the mother and baby may become fatigued and distressed during labor. A C-section is then needed to reduce the risk of harm to both the mother and the baby.

A fetus usually develops in the uterus with its head lower than its feet. In this position (called the *cephalic presentation*), the head comes along the birth canal first during delivery. Because the head is the largest part of the baby, a head-first delivery clears the way for the rest of the baby's body to slide easily out of the birth canal (fig. 1). When, as sometimes happens, the baby lies fanny first in the uterus (called a *breech presentation*), a C-section is necessary to protect the baby's health (fig. 2). The evidence for this is overwhelming. The same is true when the baby is in a *transverse position* (lying horizontally in the uterus) (fig. 3). Healthy "breech ba-

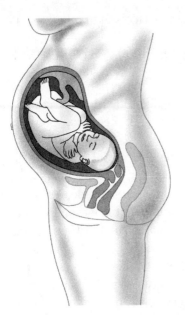

Fig. 1. Cephalic presentation

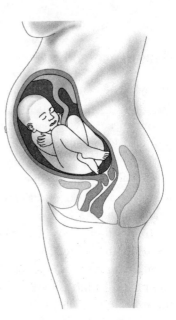

Fig. 2. Breech presentation

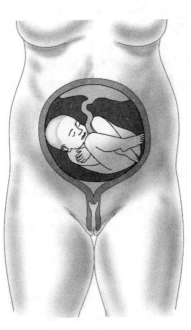

Fig. 3. Transverse presentation

bies" are delivered vaginally every day, but the vaginal delivery of a breech baby does pose greater dangers to the baby. The greatest of these dangers are that the umbilical cord will drop out of the birth canal and interfere with the baby's oxygen supply before the baby is fully delivered or that the head will not fit through the pelvis because it has not shaped itself to the birth canal. The strong muscular contractions can clamp down on the head, neck, and cord and effectively cut off all oxygen to the baby's brain. Breech births account for about 10 percent of C-sections.

Few people now argue that breech babies should be delivered vaginally. In fact, a recent study involving more than one hundred hospitals in 26 countries was halted midway through a comparison of outcomes for vaginal versus Cesarean section birth of breech babies. It quickly became obvious that C-section was a much safer way to deliver a baby lying in the breech position. The babies delivered vaginally at the beginning of this study were three times more likely to die or have birth-related injuries or disabilities than were the babies delivered by C-section.

As the mother's labor progresses, the baby's well-being is monitored by the labor nurses and the doctor. The simplest way of doing this is by intermittently checking the baby's heartbeat with a hand-held Doppler, as is done in the doctor's office. Many times, the fetal heart rate is recorded by an electronic monitor, which is placed on the mother's abdomen and held in place by an elastic strap. The monitor is connected to a printer that prints out a strip, just like an EKG. This strip is called a *cardiotocogram* or *CTG*. Sometimes a scalp electrode (which looks like a thumbtack with wires) is placed in the skin of the baby's scalp to record the heart rate. The wires from this electrode also connect to an EKG-like machine. The baby's blood-oxygen levels can also be measured by taking a drop of blood from the baby's scalp through the cervix. If the heart rate becomes abnormal or the blood oxygen becomes low, the doctor considers the baby to be "in distress" and may proceed with delivery by Cesarean section.

Ten percent of C-sections are done for nonreassuring fetal status ("fetal distress"). Electronic fetal monitoring has saved many babies' lives and preserved many babies' health by alerting doctors to the need to deliver the baby *now*. The results of this monitoring are not 100 percent accurate, however, and certainly some babies delivered by Cesarean may not have been truly distressed.

A recent advance in fetal monitoring is fetal pulse oximetry, in which a sensor is placed next to the baby's cheek in the birth canal. The sensor measures the oxygen content of the baby's blood through the skin. Although fetal pulse oximetry has improved the accuracy of diagnosing fetal distress, in studies it has not changed the number of Cesareans performed. In these studies, the diagnosis of fetal distress may have been more accurate, but there were a large number of women in the study group with a "failure" to progress in labor (see above and chap. 4). Although our methods of detecting fetal distress are not foolproof, they are the best we currently have, and it is always better to be safe than sorry. The bottom line is that the risk of delivering an impaired baby has dropped dramatically in the last one hundred years (see chap. 2). Ultimately, no mother or doctor wants to risk complications for the baby.

The remaining 20 percent of Cesarean sections in the United States are done for less common situations caused either by conditions that arise during labor or by the mother's medical condition. One condition that requires C-section delivery is *placenta previa*, where the placenta is lying partially over the birth canal and usually tears as labor begins. This tearing can cause excessive bleeding, or *hemorrhaging*. A C-section delivery is necessary with placenta previa (see chaps. 4 and 5). Hemorrhaging can also occur when the placenta is in the right place but tears abruptly in labor or even during pregnancy. Known as *abruptio placentae*, this condition is usually accompanied by severe pain. It, too, requires C-section delivery.

If a woman has an ongoing (chronic) or new (acute) medical condition that may affect her health or the baby's health, C-section delivery is often safer than a vaginal delivery. Many pregnant women with diabetes or high blood pressure, for example, are advised to plan for a Cesarean delivery. Another example is herpes infection, which can be passed on to the baby during a vaginal delivery, especially if the mother is having an active outbreak of herpes.

Preventing transmission of HIV from mother to baby is another concern. In the medical literature, doctors increasingly advocate C-section as the safest way to deliver a baby from a mother with HIV infection because Cesarean delivery helps prevent transmission of the infection to the baby. Studies done overseas of giving either one dose of Virammune (nevirapine) or a combination of Retrovir and Epivir (3TC or lamuvudine) to pregnant mothers with HIV and their babies immediately after birth showed that these treatments decrease the risk for mother-to-baby HIV transmission. In the United States several studies have shown that giving the mother Retrovir during labor and giving the baby Retrovir for six weeks starting immediately after birth will also decrease the risk of transmission. We look at these issues again in chapter 4.

C-Section: The World Experience

The world experience of C-section is not quite as one might expect. There is a great variation in rates, and the highest rates are not in the United States. The rate of Cesarean section varies from about 7 percent in some Eastern European countries and Africa to an average of 32 percent in Brazil. Among the middle and upper classes in Brazil, the rate of Cesarean birth approaches 98 percent. In that country, surgical childbirth is considered "more modern" and safer, and it has become a status symbol.

In the United States and other Western countries, about 22 percent of births are by C-section. Some people think this percentage should be lower. For example, Healthy People 2000, a consortium of government agencies and other organizations in the United States, calls for a decrease to 15 percent. As far as we can tell, the group does not explain how they arrived at that figure. We believe that the ideal number of C-sections is the one that assures that all babies at risk are safely delivered.

Unfortunately, many advocates of a specific acceptable number of C-sections arrive at a number based solely on economics. Cesarean deliveries were long thought to be more expensive than vaginal deliveries, and this is true if you consider only the cost of one procedure versus the other. Thus, the advocates for reducing C-section suggest that the largest reduction in C-sections could come from increasing the numbers of mothers who have vaginal births in subsequent pregnancies. However, we now know that a subsequent vaginal delivery is not always the most economical choice. Ultimately, it depends on whether a trial of labor ends in the vaginal delivery of a healthy baby. If it does, then there is a cost saving. However, if the trial of labor results in the vaginal birth of an impaired baby or an injury to the mother, the costs are increased. The average cost of caring for an impaired baby over its lifetime is an additional $500,000. (This figure may seem low, but you must keep in mind that the lifespan of the impaired baby may be shortened, as well.) An unsuccessful vaginal delivery is more costly than a C-section when all factors are considered. Of course, this way of analyzing the situation considers only monetary issues and ignores ethical ones.

Our sisters around the globe do not all have the luxury of criticizing high rates of Cesareans. If they had access to proper care during pregnancy and labor and the option of a timely Cesarean section, they would be spared many adverse outcomes from complications of childbirth. Obstructed labor occurs in about 5 percent of all pregnancies worldwide. It is even more common in less developed countries because women there usually have their first pregnancy in their early to mid-teens, and their pelvises are not yet fully developed. This sets the stage for great difficulty and possible tragedy, especially when you consider that proper prenatal care and modern obstetric facilities are seldom available in Africa, much of Asia, and the poorer populations of Central and South America. Many young girls labor for days, tearing their vaginas and rectums and injuring their bladders. Many babies are stillborn. Many of these young women die: for example, in Senegal, the maternal mortality rate is 0.85 percent, compared with a rate of 0.02 percent in the United States. Many others are plagued for the rest of their lives by problems such as urinary and fecal incontinence. In a recent survey of 1,348 women in the Gambia, West Africa, 46.1 percent were found to have suffered childbirth-related damage to their pelvic structures.

The Nairobi Conference in 1987 signaled the first universal action in favor of safe motherhood. Its stated objective was to decrease the number of maternal deaths by at least half within a decade. Fifteen years later, we have not begun to achieve this objective. Obstetric disorders remain the leading cause of death of women of childbearing age throughout the world. In addition, more than 40 percent of pregnant women suffer some damage or lasting disorder. The major causes of maternal mortality and morbidity in the less developed parts of the world have changed little or not at all over the past decade: hemorrhage, obstructed labor, eclampsia, infection, and abortion. Should we not be focusing our attention on fulfilling the objectives of the Nairobi Convention within our lifetimes? The accident of birth has favored those of us who live in developed countries, but we must remember our sisters in less fortunate circumstances. We must strive for reproductive health, as defined by the World Health Organization, for all women. That definition is "the ability to live through the reproductive years and beyond with reproductive choice, dignity, and successful childbearing, and free of gynecologic disease and risk."

Philosophies about C-sections and access to them vary around the world and have changed over time. Medical history provides a window onto the world of current medical practice. Before continuing with the specifics of who performs C-sections and what happens during and after the operation, we turn, in the next chapter, to the interesting history of Cesarean sections.

༄ ༄ ༄

CHAPTER 2

A Brief History of Cesarean Section

First things first: Julius Caesar was *not* born by Cesarean section! It's true that Cesarean sections have been performed for centuries, but not in the way they are performed now. Before anesthetics and antibiotics, C-sections were done only to deliver babies from dead mothers or when the labor was so obstructed that the mother and baby were surely going to die anyway.

The term *Cesarean* seems forever linked with Julius Caesar, but if he had been delivered surgically in 100 B.C., when he was born, his mother would not have lived to exchange letters with him during the Gallic war. The word *Cesarean* actually comes from the Latin word *caedere,* which means "to cut." A Roman law dating back to 715 B.C. made it illegal to bury a dead pregnant woman until the fetus had been surgically removed. Most of the babies delivered of deceased mothers were already dead, but some babies who were removed soon after the mother's death lived. An ancestor of Caesar's was probably delivered of a dead mother; such babies were referred to as *caesones.* Caesar's ancestor, a *caesone,* was named Caesar after surviving the surgical birth—and the name was passed down in the family.

From early Roman times to the nineteenth century, surgical deliveries were performed as rare and desperate measures, nearly always with fatal results for both the mother and child. However, the idea of abdominal birth reaches far back in time in many cultures. In Greek mythology, Asclepius, the god of medicine, was taken from the belly of his mother, the nymph Coronis, after she had

been executed for infidelity. Zeus tore his premature son, Dionysus, from the womb of his dead mistress, Semele, and transplanted
the baby into his own thigh, from which Dionysus was subse-
quently delivered.

In Indian legend, the Hindu god Brahma was born from a lotus
flowering out of his mother Vishnu's bellybutton. The Buddha is
said to have been delivered from the right flank of his mother,
Maya. Even Shakespeare wrote about Cesarean birth in *Macbeth*.
In the play, spirits tell Macbeth that no man born of woman will
harm him, but Macbeth later dies at the sword of Macduff, who
"was from his mother's womb untimely ripp'd."

A remarkable story of a woman surviving a C-section in 1500 is
described in an obstetrics textbook, the *Hysterotomotokie*, dated
1581. Jacob Nufer, whose wife had been in labor for many days,
implored midwives and physicians for help, but all to no avail. In
desperation, Jacob appealed to the town council and the church
for permission to try delivering his child himself. After obtaining
permission, Jacob, a swine-gelder by trade, operated on his wife.
Records indicate that his wife survived—she delivered six more
children in her lifetime, including a set of twins! A century later,
in 1610, a surgical delivery in Wittenberg, Germany, preserved the
life of both baby and mother. Unfortunately, the mother died several days later of infection. In the 1700s, Mary Donnelly helped
her neighbor Alice O'Neale of Dublin, Ireland, by delivering Alice's
baby surgically. Mary then stitched the wound with sewing thread
and dressed it with egg white. Alice survived. (The child's fate is
not revealed in the records.) Other stories of Cesarean deliveries
during the seventeenth and eighteenth centuries can be found, but
these deliveries were, undoubtedly, rare occurrences.

In the middle of the nineteenth century, successful surgery of
all kinds became more realistic with two radical advances in medicine: anesthesia and antisepsis. Some doctors and scientists were
developing anesthetics to reduce a patient's pain during surgery,
and others were starting to make connections between cleanliness
and a decrease in infection. The first advances were in anesthesia.
In the 1840s, William Morton in the United States and John Snow

in England experimented with ether and nitrous oxide (laughing gas) for both general surgery and dentistry. However, chloroform, introduced by James Simpson in Scotland in 1847, soon became the anesthetic most widely used in obstetrics. "Oh, the delightful and magical effects of it!" wrote Dr. Henry Pye Chavasse, a fashionable London obstetrician of the late 1800s. "The patient has seldom, if ever, been known to die . . . and the child when born is both lively and strong." James Simpson had to deal with the objections of clergy who claimed that trying to reduce pain in childbirth was "to contravene the devices of an All-wise Creator." Simpson cannily replied that God had put Adam into a deep sleep before removing the rib that was to become Woman and that thereby He condoned anesthesia. Queen Victoria also championed the use of anesthetics after experiencing chloroform during the delivery of one of her own babies.

Antiseptic, or sterile, surgery was a second major advance. Previously, there had been little or no regard for common cleanliness, let alone antisepsis (practices leading to the destruction of microorganisms that cause disease), in surgical wards. The surgeons and their apprentice medical students would examine a cadaver and then go directly to examine a pregnant woman without washing their bare hands. Or a doctor would perform a vaginal examination of a woman with an infection and then perform a vaginal examination to assess the progress of labor in a woman newly admitted—again, without washing his hands between examinations. This practice led to high mortality rates for vaginal deliveries as well as for surgical procedures. Women, understandably, were afraid to go to a hospital for *any* reason, including childbirth.

In the early nineteenth century, doctors who experimented with C-section mistakenly believed that there was no reason to stitch the uterine wall back together because uterine contractions would bring it together without intervention. But the actual *natural* consequence of not stitching the uterine wall back together was that many women bled to death. Along with lack of anesthetic and risk of infection, this outcome was another very good reason that C-section was attempted only as a last resort.

Joseph Lister, an Englishman working in Scotland, began experimenting with antiseptic surgery in 1865 after he became familiar with Louis Pasteur's discovery of bacteria. Lister used carbolic acid to sterilize his hands, the surgical instruments, and the catgut sutures for stitching the surgical wounds. As a result, his surgical mortality rate dropped from 45 percent to 15 percent. Even with this astounding evidence, it took nearly 30 years for "Listerism" to become common practice in surgery. Another young surgeon, William Halsted, influenced by his nurse-fiancée's allergy to carbolic acid, introduced the notion of wearing gloves during surgery, an innovation still in use. (Latex gloves, which had been used for years, in many places have been replaced by synthetic gloves because so many people in the medical environment developed latex allergy from being constantly exposed to latex dust. The purple gloves you'll see people wearing today are made of synthetic material.)

Late in the nineteenth century, in Pavia, Italy, Eduardo Porro started performing the first truly successful surgical deliveries. Porro adopted the sterile procedures of Listerism, and he also developed a unique procedure. After delivering the baby, he performed a hysterectomy and stitched the cervix, or lower part of the uterus, to the abdominal incision. The wound healed well, but of course the woman could no longer bear children. Although this must have been disappointing for some women (and perhaps a relief for others), at least they were alive and had a living baby, a fate far preferable to that of many women only a decade earlier. Like James Simpson, Porro, too, had his brush with the church: he had to obtain a special decree from the bishop acquitting him of offending public morality for contravening nature. Even so, his technique continued to be used until the early years of the twentieth century.

Surgeons soon began experimenting with closing the vertical incision in the uterus first and then closing the abdomen. Today this technique is called *classical C-section*. Surgeons discovered that both silver wire and silk made good suture materials and that infections were easier to avoid by operating early in labor, before many vaginal examinations had been done.

In 1882, Max Sanger, a German surgeon, performed 16 Cesarean deliveries, and 15 of the mothers survived—a phenomenal achievement! Cesarean surgery spread rapidly throughout Europe and the United States; at this time, most such surgeries were performed on women who had had childhood rickets or another illness that had constricted the pelvis and made vaginal delivery impossible. Many successful Cesarean surgeries were performed on women with a small pelvis or with a particularly large baby. One Scottish woman with a constricted pelvis had endured five full-term pregnancies ending in destructive operations to remove the fetus that couldn't be delivered. Her sixth baby was delivered alive by C-section. Surgeons later realized that Cesarean delivery also worked well when other obstetric complications made vaginal delivery dangerous. For example, classical C-section allowed a surgeon to scoop a baby from the uterus of a woman who had developed placenta previa, the condition in which the placenta grows over the birth canal and rips in labor. The severe bleeding in placenta previa that is often fatal to both mother and baby is avoided through Cesarean delivery.

Around 1910, surgeons began developing a technique called *lower segment transverse Cesarean section* (LSCS). In this procedure, the uterus is cut low, just above the cervix, thus decreasing the exposure of the *peritoneum* (the membrane lining the abdomen and other organs) to infection from the birth canal; by avoiding exposing the peritoneum, doctors decreased the risk of *peritonitis,* an infection of the peritoneum. It was also discovered that the lower part of the uterus actually healed better than its upper, bulbous portion. LSCS quickly replaced the classical technique for most C-section deliveries, except in women with placenta previa or abnormalities in the lower segment of the uterus.

By the jazz era of the 1920s, C-section was widely regarded as a safe procedure. Indeed, in April 1926, Queen Elizabeth II was delivered "feet first" by Cesarean. Elective, or planned, C-sections became routine when the baby was not lying in the normal head-first position and for women with small pelvises. With all deliveries in the early 1900s, little could be known about the baby's health until the baby was delivered because methods for assessing the health of the baby in the uterus were still primitive. The doctor or midwife typically poked a woman's belly, measured it with a tape measure, and listened to the baby's heart through an ear horn or with the ear directly on the belly. Thus, with early C-sections, the mother's safety remained the foremost concern.

In the early 1900s, for every two hundred pregnant women, about one died in childbirth. When a C-section was performed, that number rose to three in two hundred C-sections—which at that time seemed fairly reasonable. However, the risk to the woman increased dramatically when emergency surgical deliveries were done late in labor because infection was more likely (and antibiotics had not yet been discovered). Also, not all surgical deliveries took place in a hospital; some were done in rural areas by country doctors using laundry soap to disinfect and with inadequate light because of the fear of a flame igniting the ether.

World War I brought more advances in surgical techniques, including the ability to insert a thin tube into veins (intravenous or IV) and drip fluid slowly into a patient (the IV drip). Although doctors experimented with IVs as early as the late 1800s, this technique for replacing fluid losses, and thereby decreasing mortality from surgery, did not become sophisticated until World War I. Blood transfusion using IVs also began to be done about this time, with the help of Austrian Karl Landsteiner's 1900 discovery of the ABO blood groups. By providing obstetricians and surgeons with more options, IV techniques for replacing fluid and blood lost during delivery helped increase the safety of both vaginal and abdominal childbirth.

At about this time, the discovery and increasing use of antibiotics signaled the beginning of "scientific" medicine as we know it today. Sulfa drugs came into general use in the United States during the 1940s, but the wonder drug, penicillin, was reserved for the armed services until the latter half of the 1940s. Even in the early 1950s, the use of penicillin in the general population was still limited. Antibiotics unquestionably saved lives, but initially they were in scarce supply and were used only to treat established infections. Later, they were also administered before a C-section to help prevent infection. The effect was immediate: by 1950, fewer than 3 women in 2,000 undergoing C-section died from the operation, compared with the 3 in 200 having the surgery only a half-century before. (Now, of course, the risks are very much smaller; see chap. 6).

Since the 1950s, we have turned our sights to ensuring the health and safety of the baby in addition to that of the mother. Many techniques, including ultrasound and fetal monitoring, allow us to assess the baby's condition throughout pregnancy and delivery. With these techniques, we know when it's necessary to intervene in the delivery of a baby. Today, women need not fear that their babies won't survive or that they themselves will die in childbirth.

CHAPTER 3

ぞ ぞ ぞ

What Happens in Cesarean Section and Who Performs the Surgery?

Delphine and Ron were expecting their third child. They felt like old pros—sons Keith and Eric had been born in the birthing room in the community hospital. This pregnancy had been the easiest yet, and they were hoping that meant the baby would be a girl. Delphine was 33 years old and in excellent health. She had stayed home with the boys since Eric's birth two years earlier. She liked to say, "I'm still an early childhood educator. I'm just doing it at home now!"

In the morning, Delphine had been to see her obstetrician for her regular prenatal visit. There were still three weeks to go until her due date, and after examining her, Dr. Seip said she didn't think Delphine would deliver early because the baby's head was still high. In the afternoon, Delphine was reading to the boys while Ron cooked hamburgers. The cooking smell was making her slightly nauseous. Suddenly she felt a warm rush of fluid between her legs.

"Guess what?" she called to Ron. "My water just broke. Will you call Denise to come over for the kids and call the service to tell Dr. Seip I'm coming in? I'll grab my things."

At the hospital it was "old home week," as Delphine and Ron knew most of the staff . . . Well, in a small town, everyone knows almost everyone else! Delphine was helped into a gown while the nurses teased Ron about "being back so soon after the last one."

Sandy, the midwife from labor and delivery (L&D), appeared on the scene and closed the curtains around Delphine to examine her. She put the goop (transducing gel) on Delphine's belly and then applied the

Doppler to listen to the baby's heartbeat. And suddenly she was yelling. "Get Dr. Seip, *stat!*" The baby's heartbeat was down to 80.

Next Sandy checked Delphine vaginally and found that the cord had fallen into the vagina—a *prolapsed* cord, an obstetric emergency. Eve, one of the nurses on L&D, relayed this information to Dr. Seip by telephone. *Pandemonium reigned.* Eve relayed orders: "Get an IV in, call for an OR. Dr. Seip will be here and she wants everything ready in less than five minutes!"

Quickly, Eve and Sandy rolled Delphine over on her side on the gurney, with her knees drawn up to her chest and Sandy's hand deep in her vagina, holding the cord up. Someone else was sticking an IV in Delphine's arm and—ouch!—someone just stuck a catheter into her bladder. At the same time, the ward clerk was asking Ron to sign a consent for a C-section and the anesthesiologist was yelling at him, "Sorry, Ron, no time to explain . . . We need to get this baby out—*now.*" (In emergencies like this, one has about 20 minutes from decision to incision.)

Delphine was panicking, and she began to vomit. Just then, Dr. Seip appeared. Resting her hand on Delphine's arm, she said "Hang in there. I'll have your baby out quick as can be. Now Dr. Smith is going to put you to sleep."

By this time, they were all *running* to the operating room. Sandy clung to the side of Delphine's gurney with her hand in Delphine's vagina. Sandy could count the baby's heart rate by the pulses in the cord and was relieved that they were up to a much better 115. Delphine afterward remembered none of this because Dr. Smith had already sedated her through her IV. He had asked Ron all the questions he absolutely had to ask: Did Delphine have asthma? Did she have any false teeth? Had she ever had a high fever after surgery?

The next thing Delphine remembers vaguely is Ron telling her "Ellen is here . . . It's a girl . . . and she's beautiful . . . She has hair like a new penny . . . and she's fine." Delphine felt happy, but it was like a dream. Later she woke up in a strange room and there was Ron, holding a baby for her to see—her daughter, so pretty. But Delphine was in pain, so a nurse gave her an injection and then everything faded out again.

About eight hours later, Delphine was finally alert enough to realize that she did have her baby and that she had had a C-section. Although she was grateful that Ellen was healthy and she recognized that a tragedy had been averted, she still felt blue. Somehow she had failed with this baby—in fact, she didn't really feel like Ellen's mother yet. With the boys, she had experienced such a rush of love as soon as she heard them cry, but she hadn't even heard Ellen cry yet. She also felt guilty that she felt unhappy: shouldn't she be happy that everything turned out well?

Later still, a nurse brought Ellen in to start nursing—and wasn't that a circus! How do you hold a baby against a very sore belly? The nurse helped Delphine steady Ellen on a pillow, and Delphine watched as this little being attached herself, the long spidery fingers splayed against Delphine's breast. And then that indescribable feeling of purest love swept over Delphine.

Meanwhile, at home, Ron was feeling slightly overwhelmed at the idea of bringing home a new baby and a wife recovering from major surgery. He always took a vacation week for their baby's first week home, but Delphine would need help for longer than a week. They'd be OK next month because Delphine's mother was planning to come to help out, but for the next few weeks, things could be rough. Denise, their neighbor, came up with a good idea that saved the day. Delphine used to teach at the early childhood education center. Why not ask whether one of the college students majoring in early childhood education would like a job taking care of the two boys for the next few weeks?

Now, a year after all this took place, Delphine can tell us that she is simply full of joy with her young family. For several months after Ellen was born, however, she had a hard time, emotionally. "When I think about how hard it was for me, a woman who already had two children, I can't begin to imagine how hard a C-section must be for a first-time mother."

Delphine delivered Ellen in an emergency Cesarean section because the umbilical cord had prolapsed out of the uterus into the vagina, where it was then in a position to be compressed by Delphine's uterine contractions. As discussed in chapter 1, a C-section may be either an elective procedure or a nonelective, or emergency, procedure, like Delphine's. The surgery is the same whether the Cesarean is elective or nonelective, but the kind of anesthesia used may be determined by whether the C-section is an emergency. In this chapter we describe the surgical procedure itself as well as the options for anesthesia and the variety of health care providers you may encounter.

But first, a brief anatomy lesson.

Anatomy

Before they become pregnant and for the first few months of pregnancy, many women are unaware of their uterus, the pear-shaped organ the size of a fist that is located in the pelvis (fig. 4). It's only in about the fourth month of pregnancy that the uterus expands enough to make the belly protrude visibly. (Of course, women are also aware of their uterus if they have painful menstruation, and a uterus may be enlarged because of conditions other than pregnancy—such as uterine fibroids.)

The uterus truly resembles a pear suspended upside down in the pelvis. At the top is the rounded area called the *fundus,* and at the bottom (where the pear's stem would be) there is a narrower, pointed region, called the *cervix,* which extends into the vagina. The cervix is the uterine opening to the vagina; during labor the cervix dilates, or opens, to allow the baby to pass out of the uterus.

The uterus nestles behind the bladder and urethra and in front of the rectum in the pelvic basin. To its left and right are the waving fronds of the Fallopian tubes, each embracing an ovary. The uterus can't usually be felt by putting a hand on the belly, but a doctor can feel it when he or she does a bimanual internal exam. (In a bimanual examination, the fingers of one of the examiner's gloved hands are inside the vagina and the other hand is outside, palpating, or feeling, the organs through the lower belly wall. It is like feeling for your wallet through the walls of a handbag.) The walls of the uterus have three overlapping layers of muscle that give the uterus tremendous power to stretch and accommodate a growing baby or babies. The muscle consists of interlacing and

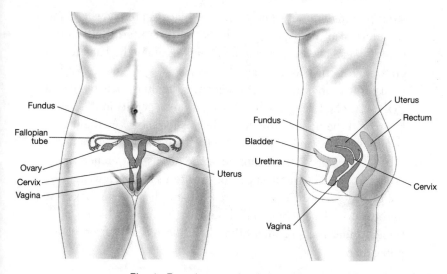

Fig. 4. Female reproductive anatomy

overlapping fibers, like a bird's nest, and has special nerves that allow it to expand to many times its size and then contract back down. (This shrinking of the uterus after birth is controlled by hormones and other factors we don't yet understand.)

During pregnancy, the uterus develops an increased supply of blood necessary for the development of the *placenta,* which nourishes the fetus. The placenta is a flattened, circular organ composed of liverlike tissue that is normally positioned at the inside upper part, or fundus, of the uterus. It is well supplied with blood, and the fetus is attached to it by the umbilical cord. (The placenta looks somewhat like a mushroom, with the stem—the umbilical cord—attached to the baby's belly.) The fetus receives nourishment and oxygen from the placenta and eliminates waste through the placenta. The placenta normally detaches from the uterus after the baby has been born, and it is delivered separately, after the baby.

The increased blood supply of pregnancy is also essential to allow the uterine muscles to contract properly during labor. The strong contractions of labor reduce the blood supply, however, and therefore also the oxygen supply, both to the uterus and to the baby. Special oxygen-carrying mechanisms allow the baby to tolerate short periods of decreased oxygen.

At three to four months of pregnancy, the uterus has increased to the size of a large grapefruit. Now, it no longer fits in the pelvic basin, and the body of the uterus begins to "show." As the uterus continues to expand, it presses on the bladder and bowels. Near the end of pregnancy, the muscle of the uterus is stretched thinly over the baby. The thinnest part of the uterus is at its lower end— the pointy end of the pear—where the baby's head or buttocks rest in the pelvis. This area is called the *lower segment,* which is positioned under the so-called bikini line, located at the top of the pubic hair.

The Surgery of C-Section

For a Cesarean section, the nurse first paints the skin of the mother's abdomen with an antiseptic solution such as Betadine (fig. 5). Next the skin is covered with drapes and sterile plastic, and the surgeon begins to make the first cut (fig. 6). The surgeon exposes the uterus by cutting through the exterior skin, through layers of fat, through the tough sheath covering the abdominal muscles, and through the peritoneum, a thin, glistening membrane lining the interior of the abdomen and pelvis (fig. 7). For a slim woman having her first C-section, this can take as little as three to five minutes. When there is more fat or when there is a previous C-section scar to cut through, this incision will take a few minutes longer. The incision may be made vertically or horizontally (see below). Once the uterus has been exposed, the surgeon begins the C-section itself.

Two types of C-section are performed: *classical C-section* and *lower segment transverse Cesarean section (LSCS)*. In classical C-section, an initial vertical (up and down) incision, about four or five inches long, is made "at the midline," in the middle of the pelvic area. This incision is made through the skin, fat, sheath covering the abdominal muscles, and the peritoneum. Once the uterus is exposed, another vertical incision is made to open the uterus (fig. 8). The classical C-section is not used very often now because the vertical incision is more likely to rupture in future pregnancies than is the horizontal incision used in lower segment transverse Cesarean section.

The LSCS is now the most commonly performed type of C-section. In the LSCS (fig. 9), an incision (again, four to five inches in length) is made through the skin, fat, sheath covering the abdominal muscles, and the peritoneum; rather than being vertical, as in the classical C-section, the incision here is made horizontally, in the shape of a curve located roughly at the top of the pubic hairline. This incision is referred to as a *Pfannenstiel incision*. Once the uterus is exposed, the lower end of the uterus is cut in the curved shape of a smile. Generally, the baby can then be lifted out of the uterus, but occasionally, if the baby is larger than expected or is lying in a difficult position and the doctor finds that he or she doesn't have enough room to get the baby out, the smile is expanded into an inverted T, with an incision running vertically up from the smile. An inverted T, like the classical incision, is more likely to rupture in future pregnancies; like the classical incision, it, too, is still used in some emergency situations.

The incision in the uterus bleeds freely while the baby is being removed, but lifting the baby usually takes only a few minutes and the uterus is stitched up right after that (figs. 10 and 11). When the uterus is stitched, the interlacing fibers of the uterine muscle contract and act as living ligatures to seal off the cut blood vessels. Most surgeons repair the incision in the uterus in two layers (fig. 12). Some surgeons, however, stitch both layers simultaneously, using an interlocking blanket stitch. The surgeon may also put in a drain, but this is optional. The drain might be used if there is much oozing from the cut surfaces, if the mother has had much previous surgery, or if there is a risk of infection. The drain is usually removed within the first week after surgery. The first few days after the surgery will be uncomfortable because C-section is major surgery and the incisions need time to heal. After surgery, the

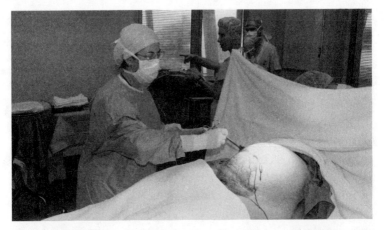

Fig. 5. Prepping the abdomen. The "prep" is an antiseptic solution that is painted on the skin. The drapes protect the surgical site from contamination by germs. Even though Jody has had three previous C-sections, she can't help feeling a little apprehensive at this stage.

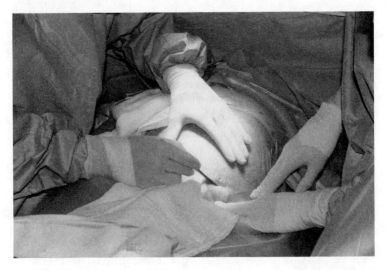

Fig. 6. About to make the incision. Jody will have a Pfannenstiel (bikini) incision low on her abdomen, right where her previous incisions were. Scars at this site nearly always heal very well.

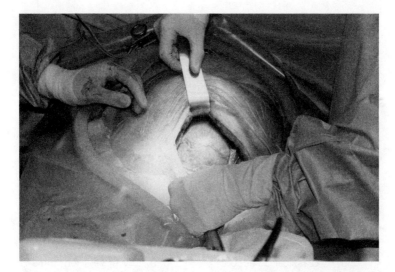

Fig. 7. The abdominal wall is opened, and the physician makes sure there is room enough to deliver the baby quickly after the uterus has been opened. In a first C-section, opening the abdomen takes only a matter of minutes, but when the woman has had C-sections or other surgeries before, opening the abdomen may take longer because the surgeon has to cut through the scar tissue that always forms on a healed incision.

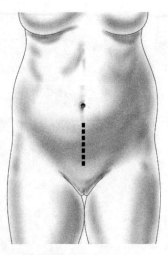 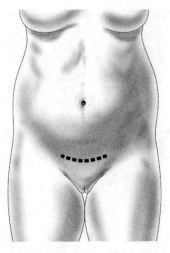

Fig. 8. Classical C-section   Fig. 9. Lower segment trans-
                                      verse Cesarean section (LSCS)

Sometimes a midline incision may be made in the skin although the incision in the uterus is transverse, and vice versa. This may be because of previous surgeries, the position of the baby, prematurity of the baby, or other reasons; the scar on the skin does not always match the scar on the uterus.

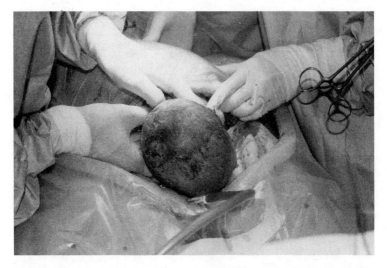

Fig. 10. Damon comes head first to peek at the world. Just as in a vaginal delivery, the head is delivered first, followed by the shoulders and then the rest of the body. The placenta is delivered just after the baby.

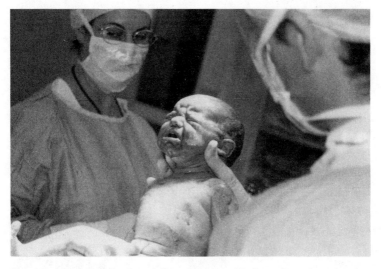

Fig. 11. Immediately after delivery, Damon is all set to protest leaving his warm nest. When the mother has had regional anesthesia, the baby is dried off, quickly checked for problems, and then handed to his parents, just like with a vaginal birth. Most doctors show the baby to the parents and let the parents see the sex of the baby even before cutting the umbilical cord.

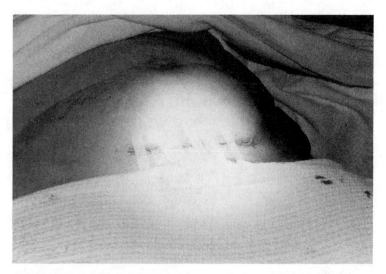

Fig. 12. All closed up. First the uterus is stitched up, and then the succeeding layers of the abdominal wall are closed. The skin may be closed by sutures or by staples.

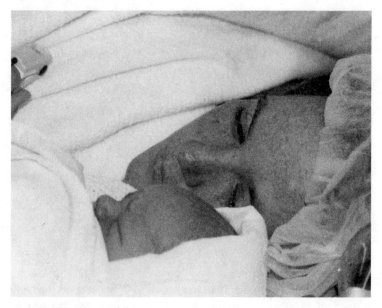

Fig. 13. Baby Damon snug in momma Jody's arms minutes after his arrival in the world via Cesarean section. Dad Clinton is nearby.

mother will have four to seven days of discomfort, possibly need-ing medication for pain. The total time for healing after C-section is about six weeks.

The uterus begins to shrink once the baby is delivered, just as in a vaginal delivery, and about six weeks after birth the uterus will be back to its prepregnancy size. For up to six weeks after birth there will also be a menstrual period–like discharge, called the *lochia,* which should taper off to light staining, if it does not stop entirely, after ten days.

Anesthesia

Like other surgeries, Cesarean sections involve anesthetizing the patient, both to keep her comfortable and so the surgeon can work quickly and effectively. Today, most anesthesia for C-sections is re-gional—either epidural or spinal anesthetic. Although general anesthesia is still used in some circumstances, regional anesthe-sia is generally safer for the mother. It allows her to be awake and lets her partner and other family members be in the room with her for the delivery. General anesthesia is used in an emergency situa-tion or when regional anesthesia is technically too difficult (usu-ally because the mother is very short or is obese) or has been tried unsuccessfully. Sometimes general anesthesia is also used for psy-chological reasons (such as extreme anxiety or fear) or for urgent medical reasons.

GENERAL ANESTHESIA

General anesthesia is most frequently used in emergency C-sections because it can be administered quickly. General anesthesia may also be used if the mother has certain medical conditions (such as previous spinal surgery), in which case a general anesthetic may be necessary or safer than regional anesthetic. General anesthesia can also be chosen for an elective C-section. The greatest concern in general anesthesia is the possibility that the mother will inhale stomach contents into the lungs *(aspiration)*. Stomach contents are acidic and can burn delicate lung tissues. Aspiration can also cause aspiration pneumonia, which is inflammation of lung tissue caused by acidic stomach contents. Treatment of aspiration pneumonia is with steroids and, in severe cases, mechanical ventilation.

If the general anesthetic is part of an elective C-section, then the mother is advised not to eat for six to eight hours before the procedure (presurgical fasting is not possible, of course, for an emergency Cesarean). Whether the Cesarean section is elective or an emergency, however, precautions are taken to avoid aspiration, even if the mother has been able to fast before the procedure. First, the mother is given antacids to decrease acidity in the stomach, and then an IV is inserted to administer fluids. Medication is put into the IV to put the mother into a light sleep. Then a tube is inserted into the windpipe (trachea) to block fluids from entering the windpipe and to funnel oxygen and anesthetic gases into the lungs. Throughout the procedure, an anesthesiologist monitors the mother and adjusts the mix of oxygen and other gases used. The mother is awakened as soon as the incision has been stitched. Although she is awake before leaving the operating room (OR), she won't remember what happens over the next few hours because of the amnesiac properties of the anesthetic.

There are some risks with general anesthesia, but less than 5 percent of women who have general anesthesia for a C-section experience problems. The most common difficulties are problems with placing the tube in the windpipe, decrease in breathing rate during the procedure, allergy to the drugs used, and a drop in blood pressure. Some women also have breathing difficulties after the operation. All of these problems respond well to treatments currently available, but they may mean a longer hospital stay and recovery period.

After general anesthesia, several steps can be taken to speed recovery and prevent pneumonia and blood clots in the lungs, the most common postsurgical complications. For example, the nurse will encourage the newly delivered woman to do deep breathing exercises, cough, and walk around the room. These exercises will cause discomfort in the patient's chest, but they are necessary for a good recovery. Wearing elastic stockings is also suggested to help prevent pooling of blood in the legs. Holding a pillow or rolled towel to the belly helps ease the pain of a cough, sneeze, or laugh.

A baby who has been delivered by C-section with general anesthesia for the mother may be a bit sleepy at first but will soon perk up.

REGIONAL ANESTHESIA

Two distinct advantages of regional anesthesia are that (1) the mother stays awake and alert for the birth and (2) she doesn't have a groggy recovery period as the anesthetic wears off, as Delphine did. For either an epidural or a spinal, the woman lies on her side or sits upright while the anesthesiologist applies a local anesthetic (like a shot of Novocain) to numb the lower back superficially (as when a cut is stitched). Then the anesthesiologist inserts a needle. For an epidural, a thin plastic tube (called a *catheter*) goes through the needle into the epidural space, located between two vertebrae and the membrane covering the spinal cord. When the tube is inserted, the woman usually feels pressure on her lower back and sometimes some tingling sensation. The anesthesiologist then administers the anesthetic through the epidural tube. After several minutes, the woman will begin to lose feeling in her lower body, as if it doesn't belong to her. During the C-section, the only feeling might be some pressure and then emptiness in the abdomen as the baby is removed. The epidural tube is left in place after the baby's delivery so the mother can control the amount of painkiller she gets. Usually, the epidural tube is removed after 24 hours, and oral medications are then used to relieve any pain or discomfort.

With a spinal anesthetic, the needle inserted in the back is much finer, and it actually pierces the membrane surrounding the spinal cord. A tube is not left in place; rather, the anesthetic is simply injected with the needle. A smaller dose of anesthetic drug is injected than with the epidural, but the numbness starts much more rapidly. Because its onset is so rapid, a spinal anesthetic, rather than a general anesthetic, can sometimes be used for unplanned C-sections that are not dire emergencies. With the spinal anesthetic, the woman may also feel the sensations of pressure and emptiness while the baby is being delivered.

The baby is safe during epidural or spinal anesthesia because the drugs are absorbed and metabolized slowly in the mother's body; this means that the baby is delivered before the drugs can even reach the placenta. Epidural anesthetics are more commonly used than spinal anesthetics because the epidural tube can be left in place after the delivery and used to deliver pain medication. Both procedures have similar risks and possible complications for the mother.

1. It may be difficult or impossible to place the catheter (epidural tube), particularly in very short or obese women. In these situations, a general anesthetic is the only other option.

2. The mother's blood pressure might drop. In this case, more fluid is administered through the IV, and the woman is sometimes turned onto her side and then turned back once the blood pressure is stable.

3. The anesthetic drugs may not take effect. This is rare but does happen for reasons that aren't well understood. In this situation, a general anesthetic must be used.

4. When the anesthesiologist inserts the needle into the back, there's a risk of nicking a vein in the epidural space and injecting some of the anesthetic drug into it. To make sure this doesn't happen, the anesthesiologist first injects only a very small amount of the drug and then monitors the heart rate and blood pressure for a few minutes and asks several questions to assess the woman's reaction. The anesthesiologist may ask, Do you feel dizzy? Do you notice a funny taste in your mouth? Do you feel any numbness of your body? The anesthesiologist is well trained to handle any problems that may arise.

5. After delivery with regional anesthetic, less than 10 percent of women experience painful headaches. These tend to result when the needle has punctured the membrane sur-

rounding the spinal cord, allowing spinal fluid to leak into the epidural space. Usually, the headache goes away with adequate fluids and lying still. However, sometimes the anesthesiologist will do a blood patch, which is a simple procedure that involves drawing some blood from the woman and injecting it into the spot where the membrane was punctured. The blood then clots and seals the hole, stopping the leaking of the spinal fluid that is causing the headache.

6. Allergies to anesthetic drugs occur very seldom, but they do occur, and they can be life threatening. The obstetrician or the woman and her family can alert the anesthesiologist to any allergies the woman or her family have. (The family history of allergies is important in part because the new baby may be allergic to the drugs.) Allergic reactions can be treated immediately by the anesthesiologist.

7. Urinary difficulties postop are not, strictly speaking, a complication of the anesthesia but of the need for a urinary catheter, although an epidural may affect the nervous control of your bladder and make it difficult to urinate for a day or two. The catheter is necessary to keep the bladder small and out of the way of being damaged during the surgery and to allow the bladder to empty automatically until the epidural effect has completely worn off. Some women develop a urinary infection because of the catheter itself, but the infection is easily treated.

8. The site of the epidural catheter may become infected, although such an infection is unusual. In case of infection, antibiotics are given; rarely, surgical drainage must be used to clear the infection.

9. Damage to the nerves coming out from the spinal column may cause some numbness and tingling in the legs or feet for up to several weeks after having the anesthetic. This feeling is strange and may be disconcerting. It usually goes away on its own after a few weeks, however. Today's sophisticated techniques for regional anesthesia have mini-

mized the risk of damage to the spinal cord and paralysis, a risk that used to be much greater.

10. Regional anesthesia may cause backache, but backache is a common problem after delivery anyway, so it is difficult to tell whether the regional anesthetic caused the backache or not. Often, backache occurs simply because the ligaments in the pelvis relax in preparation for delivery and then realign after the baby is born. Caring for an infant can, of course, also cause backache. Michele recalls: "I used to think I would be most comfortable if I just walked around bent at a 90-degree angle and never tried to straighten up. Mother's backache is in a category by itself."

As with any anesthesia, before C-section anesthesia the anesthesiologist should be familiar with your medical history and any condition you have or drug you are taking that may interfere with blood clotting. Also, if you've had prior back surgery, the anesthesiologist needs to know this information.

Obstetricians, Pediatricians, and Midwives

In the United States today, we are fortunate to have a high standard for obstetric care. Throughout your pregnancy you may see a midwife or obstetrician or family doctor for regularly scheduled prenatal visits, and that professional will also be the person who attends the delivery of your baby. Or you may encounter several different health care professionals, depending upon your health care needs. If this is your first child, then even before the baby arrives you will probably make arrangements with a pediatrician to provide care for your newborn baby once he or she arrives. You may interview several health care providers, both for you and for your baby, before deciding who will see you through pregnancy and childbirth and who will check your newborn and provide medical care for the baby. Another way to choose a health care provider is to collect the recommendations of family members or friends who have had good—or not so good—experiences. In small towns and rural areas, there may be only one provider or only a few to choose among.

If a Cesarean section is necessary, who will perform the surgery? The answer depends largely on where you are giving birth. In large medical centers in the United States, the surgery is almost always done by obstetricians—doctors with medical degrees who have completed an arduous specialized training program and have been certified by their peers as competent to perform obstetric surgeries (they then use the term *board certified* in their credentials). Sometimes a resident—a doctor-in-training—does the C-section under the close supervision of a board-certified obstetrician. In rural areas, the surgery is more likely to be done by family doctors and general surgeons who have received specific training in C-sections. There are great regional differences in large countries like the United States and Australia. In the United States, it is common for family physicians in western residency programs to be trained to do C-sections; this training is far less common in residencies in the eastern part of the country.

Today, many women choose to use a certified nurse midwife for prenatal care and delivery, and certified nurse midwives deliver many babies in uncomplicated births, usually in a hospital or birthing center and, less commonly, at home. If a C-section is necessary, an obstetrician, family physician, or general surgeon, not a midwife, performs the surgery. Many midwives continue to offer moral support after C-section but are not actively involved in the delivery. Most midwives are women, though this situation may change as more men are entering nursing in general.

Three types of midwives can be found in the United States. A *certified nurse midwife* is a fully educated and qualified nurse with specialty training in obstetrics. She is expert in uncomplicated births but knows that her training and knowledge are insufficient to handle a complicated or potentially surgical birth. Certified nurse midwives always practice with the full backup of a qualified obstetrician. Depending on the size of the hospital, the obstetrician may be in the next room, somewhere in the hospital, or within 20 minutes of arriving at the hospital once a call is placed.

Certified lay midwives are not recognized as a specialty in all states. These midwives are not medically trained; instead of attending nursing school, they learn through apprenticeship programs and demonstrate sufficient knowledge to be certified to practice in a specific state. They practice in the "wise woman" tradition, usually delivering babies at home. Their training helps them to develop a respect for the possible complications of childbirth and to realize their limits. All certified lay midwives attend births with the backup of a qualified obstetrician, which is usually a requirement of certification.

A third category is *midwives without certification.* Many of them are excellent practitioners and simply live in states that don't offer certification. We don't caution you specifically against uncertified midwives, but we do urge you to be wary of the midwife who offers no credentials, who is unable on the first visit to tell you the name of her backup physician, or who tells you that C-sections are evils to avoid. The "wise woman" tradition of acting in concert with nature is a good philosophy, but it falls down when it fails to acknowledge that sometimes a drug is better than an herb and sometimes a surgical birth is necessary.

Most of the time, in most circumstances, most health care providers are focused entirely on providing a good outcome for their patients. When a health care provider determines that a Cesarean section is necessary, the decision is always made in the interest of the health of the mother and newborn baby. Hope Roberts wrote in the *New Republic* in November 2001 about her two C-section experiences—an emergency C-section for her first child and a scheduled C-section for her second child. She concluded her piece by writing, "I chose to put my faith not in nature but in my OB-GYN, who knows all about nature's lack of concern for our happiness."

In the next chapter we look more closely at emergency Cesarean sections, which are generally performed when nature does not cooperate and a surgical procedure helps avoid a very unhappy outcome.

ֆ ֆ ֆ

When Is a Cesarean Section
an Emergency?

Michele tells the story of the delivery of her first child:

Unlike Delphine, I was a first-time mother. And I was an "elderly primip"—that unflattering term the medical profession uses for older first-timers. I was 35.

Dagobert (our in utero name for our son) was probably one of the most eagerly awaited and planned-for babies, but he was nice and cozy in my uterus and was in no hurry to leave his "nest." I had already gone three weeks past his due date and had spent daylight hours during those three weeks on the couch because of a minor elevation of blood pressure in an "old mom." *Boring.* For the previous nine months, I had worked through a mostly uncomplicated pregnancy, with, of course, my fair share of the minor maladies of pregnancy.

Then, early in the morning of October 22, 1977, I woke up to a gush of warm fluid. Even doctors don't always realize what is happening when it happens to them, and at first I thought I had wet the bed. But only for a moment.

What a funny flurry then transpired. I woke up my husband, Chris, who jumped out of bed into the nearest clothes and ran to feed the animals and start the car. Our trip to the hospital took an hour on the interstate, but I was in no discomfort. Not a twinge of labor. In fact, I never went into labor on my own. About one hour after I was admitted and had sat there with no pains or progress, a drip of Pitocin was started to induce my labor. At first very little happened, but as the doctor kept increasing the rate of drip, a crescendo of agony began to build until I felt that my middle was caught in an unremitting vise.

My first act of failure was in accepting pain meds. This baby was supposed to be spared any foreign substances, and I was determined to bear him naturally. We had even talked about home birth but decided it would not be safe at such a great distance from the hospital. But at about four or five hours into Pitocin-induced labor, I could take it no longer.

My next surrender was when I begged for a cervical block, at about 10 hours into the whole ordeal. By that time, my cervix had dilated to about five centimeters, or halfway. I was ashamed that I could not keep from crying from the pain, and I was convinced that every time I tried to breathe properly, my concentrated breathing actually brought the pain on worse. My doctor tentatively suggested a C-section, but as long as there were no signs that Dagobert was in distress, I would persevere. I had never considered the possibility of a Cesarean; after all, I was entitled to the ultimate in feminine experience: natural childbirth.

Finally, in the early hours of the 23rd, the fetal monitor indicated that Dagobert needed to come out. His heartbeat was showing changes that I, as a physician, could not ignore. My cervix was only eight centimeters dilated, so there was no way this birth could happen vaginally. At this point, great urgency informed every move, and I was whisked down the hall to the operating suite.

Twelve hours later, I held my son against me for the first time. I had a groggy memory of my husband telling me about him earlier, but I had been too sedated to be truly aware.

Although it was not the perfect birth experience that I had planned for us, our baby was (and is) perfect. He weighed eight pounds, eight and three-quarter ounces and was just too big for my five-foot frame and "elderly" ligaments. My intellect accepted the need for his Cesarean birth, but it took months for me to shake the feeling that I had failed as a woman, even though I clearly had had no other choice and it was not my fault.

In any birth there are three major elements: the birth canal, the passenger, and the force of the contractions propelling the passenger. In our case, the passenger was large and the birth canal didn't have the elasticity of a younger one. The contractions were certainly forceful, thanks to the Pitocin.

In an emergency C-section, decisions must be made relatively quickly, and often there is no time to explain the situation to the mother or prepare her emotionally for the change in plans. The attitude of the labor and delivery staff rapidly changes as they gear up from attending a woman in labor, with her own rhythm, to preparing for an emergency surgical procedure.

Some C-sections, like Delphine's, are responses to life-threatening emergencies, but probably many more are like Michele's and result from the difficulties encountered in the course of labor. These are urgent Cesarean sections, but they occur in a setting already equipped to deal with them, and there is often an indication during the labor that surgical delivery may become necessary.

As we have discussed, 70 percent of all pregnancies and labors progress uneventfully, but complications can evolve even in the healthiest and most unremarkable of pregnancies. As a consequence, we really can't accurately predict the course of any labor until the baby is delivered into the arms of his or her parents. And we must always keep in mind that the common goal of everyone involved is delivery of a healthy baby and a healthy mother. As Hope Roberts wrote in her *New Republic* piece, "I did not care about my authenticity; I cared about my baby. The only 'right way' to give birth is successfully."

We believe that every woman should have adequate knowledge about Cesareans before delivery, in case she needs to deliver by Cesarean. An elective C-section (discussed in chap. 5) doesn't carry the emotional trauma that an emergency C-section does, in part because the mother has time to come to terms with the reasons for doing the C-section. A woman having a planned Cesarean section also has time to become informed about the surgery itself. Recognizing that a C-section is a possibility in any pregnancy and understanding the possible reasons for it may make a woman feel less traumatized emotionally if her delivery suddenly becomes a surgical event, even if the decision for surgical birth is made very rapidly, to save a life or lives.

General anesthesia is used more often than regional anesthesia for emergency C-sections because general anesthesia can be quickly administered and causes the mother to lose consciousness rapidly. This is important if there are urgent conditions like hemorrhaging or prolapse of the cord or if the baby is in trouble. The mother may have rare medical problems that make a general anesthetic necessary. It is best to discuss all possible outcomes of labor with your doctor well in advance of your due date. After all, *emergency* means that we could not have anticipated this outcome. It is best to educate yourself in advance about all possibilities, including an emergency C-section and anesthesia.

At least one father, Marc, feels that fathers are left out when people talk about preparation for C-section.

Marc attended every childbirth class with his wife, Ingrid, and was excited about being her supportive coach. He had dreamed and planned for their baby just as much as she had. The morning Ingrid went into labor, Marc was beside himself. He bundled Ingrid into the car and raced for the hospital, even though he understood that first babies usually take a while.

Ingrid labored for 10 hours. Then, suddenly, her blood pressure shot up and the couple's childbirth experience turned into something you see on *ER*. Everything was happening too quickly for Marc to comprehend. All he knew was that he was scared and he was extraneous. Never before or since has he felt so helpless.

Two nurses whisked Ingrid away to the operating room while another settled Marc in an armchair in a waiting area and told him that it would be all right and that very soon he would see the baby.

After the longest half-hour of Marc's life, the nurses took him to meet his charming, red-faced daughter, Marguerite. He held his daughter and looked at her as long as the nurses let him, and then the nurse took Marguerite away to the nursery to be checked by the pediatrician.

The nurses took Marc to be with Ingrid in the recovery room, but he says he may as well have stayed outside—Ingrid was very pale and too groggy even really to know he was there. Marc felt pretty sure that Ingrid didn't know he was telling her about their daughter.

After about an hour, he realized that he was useless in there and decided to go eat something and phone all the relatives. He returned later that evening and was finally able to have his little family together.

What Marc regrets most is his belief that the trauma of the situation interfered with his bonding with his daughter. "I never felt quite as involved with her as I did with Donna, her younger sister," Marc said. Donna was also born by Cesarean, but Marc was able to be in the operating room and watch Donna be delivered.

The Reasons for Emergency C-Sections

We first discussed the "why?" of Cesarean section in chapter 1. In this chapter we provide more information about why—under what conditions—an emergency C-section may be performed: (1) conditions that occur during pregnancy and (2) conditions that occur during labor.

CONDITIONS IN PREGNANCY

Pre-eclampsia. Pre-eclampsia consists of a triad of raised blood pressure, protein spilled into the urine, and edema (fluid retention and swelling). It is more common in women who are in their first pregnancy or the first pregnancy with a new partner. We don't know why this is so or what causes pre-eclampsia. Women who have had pre-eclampsia in previous pregnancies are more likely to develop it in a subsequent pregnancy.

Blair had two pregnancies. In her first, she developed pre-eclampsia in her last trimester and had a rocky time of it. But Joanna was born vaginally, and Blair thought that the next pregnancy would be much easier. Joanna was such a delight to Blair, and two years later she got pregnant again. This time, Blair's blood pressure rose in the middle of the second trimester, and she was put to bed rest. Unfortunately, even though Blair had excellent prenatal care, at about 36 weeks of pregnancy the doctor determined that the fetus had died and that Blair would have to have a Cesarean because the fetus was lying horizontally in the uterus.

The greatest concern with pre-eclampsia is that the mother's blood pressure will get too high and she will suffer convulsions or have a stroke. Another concern is that, as happened in Blair's second pregnancy, the baby may die or be damaged by the adverse effect of pre-eclampsia on the placenta. The mother may also suffer kidney or liver damage. If a woman develops severe pre-eclampsia, her baby is safer delivered, even if very prematurely, than left in utero. This delivery often has to be done surgically because the cervix is not ready, or "ripe," for induction of labor and because labor increases the risk for convulsions, strokes, and death of the baby.

Antepartum Hemorrhage. Antepartum hemorrhage (meaning excessive loss of blood before delivery) may be caused by placenta previa, but it can also occur even when the placenta is normally positioned. Usually, the placenta is placed high up in the fundus, or ceiling, of the uterus or high on the front or back walls. In less than 1 percent of pregnancies, the placenta develops in the lower part of the uterus; this is placenta previa. The placenta's position in the lower part of the uterus in no way interferes with the supply of oxygen or nutrients to the baby or with the removal of wastes during pregnancy, but it does interfere during birth when the baby is pushed into the birth canal. And, as the lower part of the uterus starts to stretch in labor, the placenta, which is well supplied with blood, can tear. In that case, serious—indeed, fatal—bleeding can occur.

Nadine was in the last month of her fourth pregnancy and had been feeling wonderful. Sure, she was tired. Who wouldn't be, having three little ones and being as big and clumsy as a house on legs? The first morning she saw the stain on the toilet paper, she didn't think too much about it—it was so light. But when the small stain became a constant stain on her underwear and turned bright red, she knew it was time to see Dr. Green and find out what was up. When Nadine reached the clinic, she was impressed by how quickly she was whisked into the exam room. No time to catch up on the latest parents' magazines in the waiting room! Dr. Green arrived, and pretty soon Nadine was off having an ultrasound. She had refused earlier requests that she have an ultrasound.

Half an hour later, Nadine's husband, Ben, had arrived at Dr. Green's office, and Dr. Green was telling the couple that the placenta was lying across the birth canal and that the only safe way to deliver this baby was by Cesarean. Nadine and Ben were stunned, but as Dr. Green explained more about the situation, they were able to accept the necessity for the surgery. Nadine was given some medications to help the baby's lungs mature and told to stay in bed for several days. The hope was that the surgery could be delayed until the next week, but no, the bleeding got heavier over the next day. The C-section was quickly done, and Brett was born—a little early but as healthy as could be.

Sometimes, bleeding will occur from a normally positioned placenta, for reasons that we don't understand. If the bleeding is heavy or persistent, a Cesarean delivery is the safest choice then, too, for the health of the baby.

Medical Conditions in the Mother or Retarded Growth of the Fetus. When the expectant mother has a specific medical condition, such as diabetes or hypertension, that might affect the pregnancy or birth, her health and the growth of the fetus are carefully monitored. Generally, the decision between a surgical delivery and a closely monitored vaginal delivery is made by the parents and their doctors over the course of weeks, before labor begins, rather than more urgently, during labor. If, during routine prenatal visits, it becomes obvious that the fetus is not growing as it should, either close and careful monitoring will continue or an emergency C-section will be done. That's what happened with Latisha.

Latisha considered herself a very healthy woman. True, she had been diagnosed with high blood pressure, but the condition had responded well to medication, and she hardly gave it thought. She and her partner, Christopher, had waited until now—her 35th year—to start a family because they wanted first to have a house and some savings in the bank. Never, ever did she think of herself as having a condition that could complicate her pregnancy.

The pregnancy was most uneventful until Latisha's 34-week checkup. The tape measure showed no increase in her belly since the last visit, two weeks earlier. It seemed that the baby had stopped growing. Dr. Owens ordered CTGs three times during the next week, to monitor the growth of the baby. A CTG, or cardiotocogram, is a monitoring of the baby's heart, an in utero EKG. The third CTG showed a very abnormal heart rate. Much to Latisha's surprise, she was whisked off to the OR, and 15 minutes later Martin was delivered by Cesarean. He needed special care at first and spent his first few days in the neonatal special care nursery, but he is now a healthy eight-month-old.

Maternal Infection. Some maternal infections require close monitoring during pregnancy and delivery to prevent transmission of the infection to the baby. The best known of these infections is vaginal herpes. If a woman has an active vaginal herpes outbreak when it is time for her baby to be born, a C-section may be necessary to protect the baby from infection. Women with a history of vaginal herpes need to be aware of this possibility.

As discussed in chapter 1, maternal HIV infection is more than adequate reason for a C-section delivery. Usually, the woman would know she was going to deliver by Cesarean, but the infection may not be discovered until labor begins in a woman who has not had prenatal care. In that case, the surgery would not be anticipated. Another option when the mother is HIV positive is to allow vaginal delivery to proceed after giving the mother either a single dose of Virammune or a combination of Retrovir and Epivir before delivery; the baby is given a single dose of Virammune or is treated with Retrovir and Epivir within 72 hours of birth. This approach is not 100 percent effective, however.

CONDITIONS IN LABOR

Failure to Progress in Labor. This is what happened with Michele, whose story opened this chapter. It is most common in first-time mothers and often occurs because of the position of the "passenger" in the birth canal. That is, progress of labor can be affected by how the fetus's head is positioned in the birth canal and whether the head flexes down in the chin-to-chest position adequately to allow the baby to be pushed through the birth canal. Failure to progress in labor often can be managed by giving the mother intravenous *Pitocin* (a synthetic form of *oxytocin,* which is a pituitary hormone that stimulates the uterus to contract), as was done with Michele. Stimulating contractions with Pitocin is called *active management of labor.* The Pitocin affects the force and rhythm of the uterine contractions, and these more powerful contractions can sometimes effectively "persuade" the passenger to move along in the birth canal.

As is illustrated by Michele's story, however, active management of labor is not always effective. And doctors know from bitter experience over the years that, if labor is too long, fetal distress can develop and the baby can die or sustain birth injuries. If you think of the strong forces that are consistently and repetitively exerted on the fetus in labor, with little or no relief, the possibility for fetal distress in a long labor certainly makes sense.

It also makes common sense, and is borne out by experience, that the mother may be injured by prolonged labor. She may, for example, develop a *fistula,* which is a tear (or passage) into a nearby space, most commonly the rectum or the urethra. Formation of fistulae in labor is so common in the developing world that it has been the subject of international conferences. (In Ethiopia, a specialized fistula hospital exists just to repair the damage suffered by women in childbirth. And this hospital is able to accommodate only a very small percentage of the women who are affected by childbirth-related fistulae.) A fistula must be surgically corrected, or the woman may leak feces and urine for the rest of her life and have recurring vaginal infections because there is an open connection between the vagina and the rectum or the vagina and the bladder. In the developed world, few women develop a fistula in childbirth, largely because C-section is widely available and is used when necessary to avoid such complications of birth.

Nonreassuring Fetal Status. Fetal distress often occurs when labor fails to progress. Contractions of the uterus in labor reduce the blood supply to the fetus and therefore reduce the fetus's oxygen supply. This situation can be tolerated by a healthy baby for the brief rhythmic periods associated with labor over a limited time. If the fetus is already having difficulties of any kind, however, he or she may suffer from lack of oxygen, and the level of acidity in his or her blood will rise. Doctors are able to monitor the baby's heart rate, either on a fetal monitor or by frequent checks by trained birth attendants. If the fetus is in trouble, the heart rate will drop. The most current terminology states that the heart rate is "nonreassuring." The normal heart rate for a fetus or newborn baby is 120 to 160 beats per minute—much higher than an adult's. Any sustained drop below that range is cause for concern and probably for immediate delivery.

The acidity of the baby's blood can be measured by taking a sample of the baby's scalp blood, as long as the mother's cervix is dilated enough to allow a sample to be taken. This is safe for the baby. If the blood is acidic, then immediate delivery is necessary. If the baby's heart rate drops but the blood does not become acidic, then it may be safe to continue labor, monitoring very closely, and avoid C-section. As noted in chapter 1, a new advance in checking fetal status is fetal pulse oximetry, in which a small gadget is placed in the vagina, next to the baby's cheek. This gadget measures the oxygen in the baby's blood.

Cord Prolapse. This is what happened with Delphine (chap. 3). The cord may fall into the birth canal if there is room for the cord to slip past the baby into the birth canal; this situation is most common in breech (bottom-first) or transverse (lying horizontally) presentations of the baby, but it can also happen if the baby's head has not settled down into the birth canal (has not *engaged*). When the uterine waters break, the cord may slip out. A prolapsed cord is a life-threatening emergency for the baby, who must be delivered by C-section.

Hemorrhage during Labor. Michele recounts,

One night, when I was a resident, I wandered into L&D to use their toaster. It was very quiet in there—not their usual bustle. Soon, it was apparent that everyone was tied up with simultaneous deliveries, so when a young woman in labor room 3 asked me for a bedpan, I brought it to her. After I finished my toast and peanut butter, I went back to take the pan from her. To my horror, I found the pan was full of blood, and this woman was bleeding heavily. I opened her IV to full volume and yelled for help. Within 20 minutes, her baby greeted the world. Because of the unusually busy night, all necessary staff were not only in the hospital but actually in the labor and delivery department. As they say, it must have been either a full moon or a thunderstorm!

This mother's placenta was low-lying, but there had been no hint of impending difficulties during her pregnancy. Sometimes the placenta is situated at the top of the uterus in a normal position but separates from the uterus prematurely (before the baby is delivered) and bleeds. Whatever the specific cause of excessive bleeding during labor, the baby must be delivered urgently by C-section because the hemorrhaging threatens the lives of both baby and mother.

Severe Hypertension, Pre-eclampsia, or Eclampsia during Labor. Any of these conditions can be truly frightening for both mother and doctor. These conditions can cause convulsions, stroke, or liver or kidney failure in the mother, and urgent delivery is necessary, usually by C-section.

During medical school, both Caroline and Michele knew Brenda, the wife of a fellow student. Brenda was pregnant with their first child and had had a reasonably uneventful pregnancy. Labor began normally, but suddenly, in the second hour of labor, Brenda's blood pressure rocketed up and she had a major seizure. She was stabilized with medications and whisked off to the OR. Happily, both Brenda and her son survived that experience in good shape.

Monitoring the condition of the mother during labor, of course, is essential. Careful monitoring alerts the health care team to any developing problems that may affect the mother's health in the short term and long term.

Other Maternal Disease Worsening during Labor. Many medical conditions, including heart disease, pulmonary hypertension, and diabetes, can potentially compromise a woman's ability to handle the extreme physical stress of labor and delivery. A woman may have a problem, either congenital or acquired, affecting her pelvis in such a way that makes vaginal birth impossible. Any of these conditions may make a C-section the safer choice, and the C-section will be performed urgently if these conditions are discovered or become worse during labor.

Nonemergency C-sections, discussed in the next chapter, may be performed for some of the reasons described in this chapter, but they are planned ahead.

CHAPTER 5

ॐ ॐ ॐ

When Is a Cesarean Section Not an Emergency?

Emily and John, both 37 years old, had prepared very carefully for parenthood, and with the biological clock ticking away, the couple began trying to conceive a baby—but without success. Soon they found out that Emily had endometriosis (an overgrowth of tissue around her tubes and uterus)—placing a huge hurdle in the way. Emily and John were seriously considering in vitro fertilization. In fact, they had decided that in three months, after Emily completed a major project at work, they would go for it.

A few weeks later, Emily and John were enjoying a Sunday brunch when Emily was overcome by waves of nausea. She felt so bad she had to go home and spend a few hours lying down. Must be a nasty bug, she thought.

But this "bug" kept affecting her every morning and being cured by noon. Finally, Emily's secretary asked her, "Emily, do you think you might be pregnant? This is very much like morning sickness."

"You're right!" Emily said, "I never thought of that." And she was off to the pharmacy for a home pregnancy test. She and John were full of joy when the result showed she was, indeed, expecting. Because of Emily's age and endometriosis, her doctor thought that Emily would be best served by the university hospital in the next town, the same hospital she would have gone to for in vitro fertilization. It was not inconvenient and both John and Emily felt very comfortable with Dr. Wu, at the university hospital.

Things were pretty uneventful and the morning sickness subsided. At 16 weeks of pregnancy, Emily had an amniocentesis because of the increased risk of the fetus having Down syndrome at her age. All was OK. She and John had felt very conflicted about what to do if the fetus had an abnormality, but, fortunately, no decisions had to be made. They opted not to know whether it was a boy or a girl; they had given the baby an in utero name of Ivy.

The rest of the pregnancy went boringly well until, at 32 weeks, Dr. Wu told them the baby was in a breech position. She wasn't overly concerned at this point because there was still time and room for the baby to turn, but she advised that they should do an ultrasound in a few weeks and get a look at things.

At 36 weeks, Ivy was still in a breech position and Dr. Wu offered to try turning the baby—a maneuver called *external cephalic version* (ECV). To perform the maneuver, the doctor uses her hands on the pregnant belly to try to push the baby into a different position. ECV has some risks (for example, tightening the cord around the fetus's neck or tearing the placenta), and very often the baby slips back into the original position. The few good studies of ECV that have been done report only about a 40 percent success rate. Because of the possible risks associated with this procedure, it should be attempted only by a well-trained physician.

Emily and John didn't want to take any risks with Ivy, so, after a lengthy discussion of risks versus benefits, they decided that, if Ivy stayed breech, they would have an elective C-section. They toured the delivery wing of the hospital and signed all the necessary papers. They also met with the anesthesiologist, and Emily had blood work done, including blood typing, in case blood should be needed during the surgery. (Blood transfusion during C-section is unusual, but it is best to be prepared for all possibilities.) A date was scheduled for Ivy's birthday.

Day 1. At last, the day arrived. All the tests showed that Ivy was mature enough to be born, but that he or she still wanted to "back into" life, so plans for the C-section were made. Emily entered the hospital early in the morning, without breakfast, and was shown to the showers. After showering, she put on a hospital gown (sometimes called a "johnny") and paper slippers and pushed her hair up into a paper cap. She draped the hospital dressing gown to conceal her bare back. After the delivery, she was told, she could wear her own clothes, but for now she had to use these.

Back in her room (truly a little cubicle but private, at least), Emily was visited by a nurse who shaved the top two inches of her pubic hair. Next an IV technician arrived to put in an IV. Then the worst indignity so far: the nurse inserted a urinary catheter, explaining that it is necessary so the bladder would not be full and in danger of being nicked. Emily was glad the nurse was a woman.

John rejoined Emily as the nurse directed her to hop up (she must have been kidding!) on the gurney, and it was off to the OR. At this point, Emily began to feel a little panicky. John held her hand and kept reassuring her.

In the OR, Dr. Edwards, the anesthesiologist, had Emily curl up on her side in a fetal position. It felt like her belly was pushing through her throat. She then felt the cold of the antiseptic swabbing her back and then a sting. Next there was a weird pressure sensation and electricity down one leg: Dr. Edwards said "Sorry," so that "lightning" sensation must not have been in the plan. The epidural was in and she was turned onto her back.

Over the next few minutes, Emily felt her whole lower abdomen and back turn very cool and numb. Then Dr. Edwards asked, "Do you feel this?" She didn't. In fact, by now her whole lower body felt like some leaden and improbable appendage, not a real part of her.

Apparently some sort of signal was given because then the OR became a hive of activity. Dr. Wu was there, and John was there, sitting beside Dr. Edwards, by Emily's head, and holding her hand. Then it felt like Dr. Wu was drawing on Emily's belly—how strange—followed by a tugging and pulling sensation and a weird empty feeling and then a baby's cry. "Emily, say hello to your son."

Dr. Wu handed the baby to John, who held him so that Emily could see him and then handed him to Dr. Mayer, their pediatrician, to check over. Ivy was now Ethan. Because the OR was too cool, Dr. Mayer took Ethan to the nursery. John went with them, while Emily was being "done up." It didn't take long. (When Emily looked down at her belly later, the staples made her think of braces on teeth.)

After a brief stay in the recovery area, Emily was back in her room. John watched with tears in his eyes as Emily put Ethan to her breast, and he latched on as though he'd been doing this forever. At this moment, Emily realized for the first time how absolutely pooped she was! So this is why the hospital won't allow visitors the first day! Now it made all the sense in the world. John returned Ethan to his Isolette, put him where Emily could see him, and went to phone the world (somewhere out of the room, so Emily could sleep).

Day 2. The next day Emily was freed of both the IV and the catheter. Such relief! She ate a boring diet of tea, toast, and Jello, enlivened later in the day by some broth and mashed potato. Her first shower felt like heaven, but she was glad the nurse was there because she felt slightly woozy. That evening, she had a small bowel movement and rang to tell the nurse: she knew a BM meant she could have real food! That night Ethan stayed in the room with her.

Day 3. Real food and an appetite. Her belly was sore, but it was OK if she avoided laughing and held a pillow to it when she walked. Cradling Ethan on a pillow to nurse worked very well, too. Once in a while the pain pills were welcome, but they made her drowsy, and she didn't want to miss a minute of this miracle who is her son. John worked these two days so he could take a week off when she and Ethan got home.

Surprise, surprise! That evening Dr. Wu came around and told Emily that, because she was doing so well, she could go home. Initially she was delighted, but then she realized that she would have no help at home until the following evening, when her mother would arrive and John could take off work. So, the plan was made: day 4 it is.

Day 4. Emily was glad she'd stayed because already on day 4 she was able to shower by herself and walk the halls without being woozy. Truth to tell, she had felt a little frightened about going home. Now, Mom and John would both be there. The nurse took out some of the staples and gave Emily an appointment card for the following Monday to see Dr. Wu so the rest of the staples could be removed. There was also an appointment card for Ethan to have a two-week checkup with Dr. Mayer.

The Reasons for Elective C-section

MALPRESENTATION

The "presentation" is the part of the baby that greets the world first. As we discussed in chapter 1, the normal presentation is head first. Head first is the most common presentation and is the safest way for the baby. The head is the largest part of the baby and, once it successfully navigates the birth canal, the rest of the baby usually just slithers out. The skull is still soft and malleable at this stage, so it can change shape in the birth canal without damaging the baby's brain.

About 4 percent of babies present feet or bottom first in a breech presentation. The danger in a breech is that the body—the smaller, softer parts of the baby—will easily deliver, and the umbilical cord with them, but the head may get hung up. This cuts off oxygen to the brain and the baby may die or be seriously damaged. In a woman who has already delivered one or more babies vaginally—especially if they weighed seven or more pounds—the risk of damage is decreased because, in a sense, we know the track record of her birth canal. In a woman like Emily, who has never delivered a baby vaginally, however, we are very afraid for the breech baby, and a C-section is the clear medical choice. There have been several studies analyzing breech births, and the international consensus is that C-section is the preferred method of birth for a breech baby.

Other presentations are much more unusual, but sometimes a baby will decide to reach out for the world with a fist or shoulder. This just doesn't work! If these babies don't turn, a C-section will be necessary to deliver them safely.

As noted in Emily's story, doctors sometimes try to turn a baby from the outside of the mother's body, in a procedure called external cephalic version. In this procedure, the attempt is made to turn the baby from his breech or other unusual position to a head-first, or cephalic, position, so his or her head will enter the birth canal first. ECV is done by putting gentle but firm pressure on the mother's belly and attempting to push the baby into the desired position. The baby's heartbeat has to be monitored carefully while the procedure is done. There is little scientific evidence about how often and how well ECV works, and sometimes babies who have been successfully encouraged into a head-first position flip back into breech. The procedure carries some risks, too. The placenta may tear, or the umbilical cord may become entangled or compressed, causing fetal distress that could make an urgent C-section necessary or maybe even cause the baby to die. This procedure should not be attempted lightly or by nonexpert hands.

Sometimes nature takes over, as Trudy's story demonstrates.

Trudy's first baby, Stella, was born by C-section because she was in a breech presentation. Her obstetrician had tried to turn the baby, but the procedure didn't work, so Stella was born by scheduled C-section. In Trudy's second pregnancy, Trudy wanted to try a vaginal birth, but in the last trimester this baby, too, was in a breech position. Her doctor didn't dare try to turn this baby because the scar from the previous C-section might cause the uterus to rupture. A second C-section was scheduled.

One week to the day before the scheduled surgical birthday, Trudy arrived at the hospital in active labor. Baby Sam had turned himself around! Only six hours later, his healthy yell greeted the world. Trudy delivered Sam into the capable hands of a certified nurse midwife.

REPEAT CESAREAN SECTIONS

By far the most common reason for a C-section is that the woman has had a previous C-section. When Michele was pregnant with her second child, she knew that she had the choice of a "trial of labor" or a repeat C-section. "By this time, I had gotten over my preconceived notions of the desirable way to have a baby," she recalls, "and there was no way I would go through that agony again. I liked the idea of a nice, calm, *planned* C-section. I also knew that my recovery would be much quicker for not having those exhausting hours of labor. I noted with interest that women who questioned my decision had all had brief and uneventful deliveries. To each her own!"

Michele's aunt had seven children. They were born in the 1940s and 1950s, and after the first two, all were C-sections. In those days, it was automatic: once a woman had one C-section, all later babies would be delivered by section. This rule was in place because there was real concern that during labor the uterus would rupture along the previous Cesarean scar. Aunt Bettye had broken another rule of the time, which said it was only safe to have two or three C-sections—again, because of the fear that the scar would not hold. Like Michele and her aunt, many women have viewed their scars like zippers for popping out their little ones.

Today the prevailing medical wisdom is that many women can have a trial of labor after having had a previous C-section. This means exactly what it says: with a doctor's approval, a woman can try to go through labor and deliver vaginally *if she wants to*. For any woman who decides to have a trial of labor, an operating room is prepared and waiting in case the trial is deemed unsafe to continue and she needs a C-section. No woman has to have a trial of labor if she doesn't want to.

Repeat C-sections are recommended in the following circumstances:

- when the reason for the previous section is still present—for example, when a woman's pelvis is misshapen and narrow from a childhood accident
- for women who have had a previous classical C-section (cut up the front of the body of the uterus) or similar surgery on the uterus
- for women who have had three or more previous C-sections (in practice, usually women who have had two or more)
- for women who do not want to attempt a trial of labor

These are accepted guidelines in all countries. We discuss all of these circumstances in more depth in chapter 10, on vaginal birth after C-section.

MEDICAL CONDITIONS IN THE MOTHER

A woman with hard-to-control diabetes, longstanding high blood pressure or a history of stroke, HIV infection, or many other less common medical conditions may be advised to have an elective C-section for her own and her baby's health. For example, the exhausting physical exertion of labor may pose serious risks to a woman with cardiac illness—and to her baby.

Some gynecological conditions, such as a large fibroid or an ovarian cyst, may act as a roadblock to the passage of the baby down the birth canal. Often under these circumstances a C-section is necessary to deliver the baby. (A *fibroid* is a tumor, a mass of muscle in the uterine wall, similar to a knot in a pine board.)

An elective C-section may also be suggested to an older woman who has finally gotten pregnant after years of infertility. All babies are precious, but the reasoning here is that perhaps this woman couldn't become pregnant again if anything went wrong, so it is imperative that this pregnancy have a successful outcome. These words appear harsh even as we write them, but the reasoning is sound and is based on obstetric experience.

If you have medical reasons for having an elective C-section, sit down with your doctor and thoroughly discuss your medical condition and why a C-section is necessary for you.

PLACENTA PREVIA

As we discussed in chapter 4, a placenta previa is a placenta that is positioned, for the most part, over the cervix. As the uterus contracts and the cervix dilates to allow the baby to pass through, the placenta is torn away from its attachment to the uterus. The progression of the labor only makes matters worse. This is an uncommon condition but one that almost always requires a C-section, as we saw with Nadine. In most cases today, placenta previa is diagnosed through ultrasound examination early in a pregnancy, before any bleeding occurs. No one wants to take any chance of hemorrhage at all, so a C-section is absolutely the best choice when placenta previa is diagnosed. (Sometimes, as we have seen, placenta previa is not diagnosed until bleeding occurs, and in that case the Cesarean is not an elective procedure but an emergency.)

The Advantages of Elective Cesarean

What are the advantages of a planned C-section over an emergency? Obviously, you have more time to think about it, ask questions about it, and adjust to the idea of it. You can also arrange a support system: your parents, siblings, and friends know in advance when their help will be needed. This is especially important if you are going home to other small children. (We'll talk more about this in chap. 7, on what to expect and how to cope when you go home.) The night before delivery, you may want to have a small get-together with friends or an intimate dinner with your partner (just don't overdo on food and drink or get overtired).

In most emergency C-sections, general anesthesia is used because it can be administered quickly. With a planned C-section, the mother often can choose which type of anesthetic she wants. Although some women who are having a planned C-section prefer a general anesthetic, most women don't want to miss the conscious experience of their baby's birth, and they choose regional anesthetic. Another advantage of planned C-section is that, if you are having general anesthesia, you can fast (not eat anything for 12 hours) before the procedure, so aspiration is less of a concern than it is in emergency C-section.

The following two stories demonstrate some of the reasons for choosing general anesthesia over local anesthesia and vice versa (these forms of anesthesia are described in detail in chap. 3). Generally, the decision about type of anesthesia is dictated by the mother-to-be's medical condition and that of her baby. To a lesser, but important, degree, it is also determined by the mother's preferences, which will be honored if there is no medical reason not to do so.

Olga was 42 when she first became pregnant. Her partner, Hiro, was in his fifties and already had a grown first family. Neither of them had expected to fall in love, let alone find themselves about to be parents.

In the last weeks of Olga's pregnancy, her blood pressure began to rise, and it was clear to her obstetrician that her uterus would not respond to induction of labor, so an elective C-section was suggested. Olga felt panicked; she had never been in a hospital and was afraid she couldn't handle being in an OR. It didn't help that Hiro was even more apprehensive.

Although a general anesthetic is not the preferred choice for an elective C-section, after Olga had heard about all the procedures and risks, she suggested and everyone involved agreed that, for her, a general anesthetic might be the better way to go. Olga entered the operating room on the gurney, an IV line was inserted, and the anesthesiologist told her that he was going to place a mask over her nose. The anesthetic gas would be mixed with oxygen, and she would quietly breathe it. She might be aware of a little pressure on her neck as she fell asleep. This feeling should not alarm her, as it was simply the tube being placed in her throat to deliver gas directly to the lungs and protect her from inhaling any vomit.

In fact, all Olga remembered was gently falling asleep. Her next memory was a hazy one of Hiro telling her they had a beautiful daughter. Later that day, she came fully awake and was able to hold her little Anna.

Renee approached her impending C-section with the sang-froid of youth. She was 23 and had been very happily married to Tony, also 23, for a year. Both of them were in the best of health and fitness and had accepted the breech presentation of their baby and the necessity of a C-section delivery as "one of those things."

Renee had opted for an epidural anesthetic, partly for medical reasons but mostly because she wanted to be awake for the birth of her baby and wanted to see Tony's face. He planned to be with her throughout the delivery. To prepare, they had watched a video of a Cesarean birth from their doctor.

Finally, the delivery date arrived. Renee and Tony went to the hospital at about eight in the morning and were shown to a small cubicle, where Renee changed to a hospital gown. In another room, the anesthesiologist explained everything she was going to do. Next Renee was instructed to curl up around this basketball that used to be her lap, and then she felt a cold wash on her lower back. There was a small sting as the local anesthetic was injected to numb the skin of her lower back where the needle was going.

The anesthesiologist inserted a thin plastic tube through a disposable needle into the space between the bone of the vertebrae and the membrane covering the spinal cord—the epidural space. Renee experienced this as a hard pressure on her low back and a few transient tingling sensations. After several minutes, she had the very strange feeling of "losing her legs." The anesthesiologist had injected local anesthetic through the catheter (tube), and Renee's skin from her bellybutton down was growing numb.

Renee was helped onto her back and Tony took her hand. Although she wasn't aware of this, the anesthesiologist mixed a painkiller in with the local anesthetic to help make sure she was comfortable during and after the C-section. They wheeled Renee into the OR, Tony staunchly by her side, where her obstetrician was waiting. Within about five minutes, he had made the cut into her abdomen—which hardly felt like anything at all. Then, when he was taking the baby out, Renee was aware for a few minutes of an unpleasant pressure sensation followed by the strangest feeling of emptiness. For just a second or two she felt faint, but the feeling passed as their daughter was held up to meet her Momma and Poppa. Such a melting joy when she heard Felicia cry. Tony went with the baby and the pediatrician to count toes while Renee was stitched. Half an hour later they met again in the recovery area.

For the next 24 hours, Renee was able to control her pain by using self-administered medication through the epidural catheter, which had been left in place for that purpose. By pushing a button, she could release a controlled amount of painkiller into the tube in her back. Once the epidural catheter had been removed, her discomfort was adequately controlled with oral medications.

Michele also had epidural anesthesia for her second C-section and found it made the second surgery much easier. For one thing, she wasn't knocked out for more than half a day afterward, and she was able to hold and nurse her second child much more quickly than she had her first. Also, she was able to enjoy a visit from her two-year-old on the same day and introduce him to his new sister. "Sure, I hurt and I was tired," she recalls, "but it wasn't the same bone-drained fatigue that I had experienced after labor followed by general anesthetic."

All the way around, a planned C-section is by far less stressful and less hurried than an emergency one, which means there are fewer chances for something to go wrong. You know the date ahead of time and can plan ahead. You may be able to choose your anesthetic. You are not exhausted from labor afterward. And, should you go into labor before your "appointment," a C-section can still be performed, usually with little difference other than experiencing labor pains and having the baby on a different date.

Because there is so much overlap between the reasons for emergency and the reasons for planned C-sections, the differences between them can be confusing. In fact, the reasons for having a Cesarean are the same in both situations, but the urgency differs. When the reason is known ahead of time (for example, a breech presentation), a C-section can be planned; if the reason (for example, nonreassuring fetal status) is not known until the woman is in labor, surgery becomes urgent. And, as we have seen, a planned C-section may become more urgent if the mother unexpectedly goes into labor.

CHAPTER 6

✧ ✧ ✧

Considering the Risks of Cesarean Section

Without surgical intervention during delivery, many a mother's or infant's health would be harmed or their lives put in danger. As we have seen in our own practices and as we have related in the stories in this book, C-sections have saved the lives of many, many women and infants and have prevented much injury and disability. C-sections offer the blessings of health and life. Nevertheless, we should not lose sight of the fact that a Cesarean section is major surgery: a C-section involves opening the abdomen and (after moving the bladder out of the way) cutting into the uterus, working near some major blood vessels and sometimes having to push the blood-rich placenta out of the way. Like any surgery, even minor surgery, C-section carries some risk.

We devote this chapter to a discussion of these risks. We do so not to alarm you but (as with the rest of the information in this book) to inform you. A woman who understands what happens in C-section (see chap. 3), including the risks of the surgery, will be better equipped to understand and cope with any problems that may develop during or after the surgery. Some of the complications of surgery occur during the procedure, and others show up in the first 24 to 36 hours after surgery. It is important to put these risks into perspective—that is, to be able to weigh the risks of surgery and the risks of delivering vaginally and come to the conclusion that the surgery is or was necessary for all the reasons discussed in earlier chapters.

Most C-sections are performed because of difficulties with the mother's health or the health of the baby; any significant medical problem in itself carries a certain amount of risk. For example, severe hemorrhage is more often associated with Cesareans than with vaginal deliveries, but this is understandable when we consider that severe hemorrhage can occur because of placenta previa or placental abruption, which are *treated* by C-section. These conditions cause bleeding before birth (antepartum hemorrhage; see chap. 4) and are associated with bleeding after birth, as well. The reason is twofold; these conditions interfere with the normal mechanisms that, first, make the uterus contract down and, second, clamp closed the vessels that bleed from the site of the placenta. Also, these conditions can interfere with the normal clotting mechanisms of the blood. When a woman develops a condition that causes bleeding and interferes with healing, she is more likely to suffer severe hemorrhage. There is little to be gained by comparing her outcome with the outcome (or the amount of bleeding) of a straightforward vaginal delivery, free of complication.

In C-section, as in all operations, the *risk* of doing the surgery must be balanced against the *reason* for doing the surgery. Consider the C-section performed for a breech presentation, for example. Here, the risks to the mother from the surgery are minimal, but the risks to the baby from vaginal delivery are significant. These risks include severe brain damage and death. These are intolerable risks, and they are real risks: properly conducted medical trials have confirmed this, as we discussed in chapter 1. In saying this we are not saying that all breech babies delivered vaginally will be harmed, but we are saying that it is statistically safer to deliver breech babies by C-section than by vaginal delivery. And we know that when it is your baby we are talking about, statistics matter even more.

Before we turn to the specific risks of C-section, a caveat is in order. Most of the studies described in the literature lump all C-sections together when measuring risks. This means that the outcomes of C-sections done for placenta previa or on women who have had previous Cesareans are considered right along with the outcomes of Cesareans done as planned procedures for breech presentation. Common sense tells us that the risks associated with these different situations differ. Risk figures for uncomplicated, planned C-sections in healthy women are hard to find. If you are planning a Cesarean birth, you will want to discuss your own specific risks with your physician.

The risks of Cesarean section are the same as those of any surgery:

- the risks of anesthesia
- bleeding, either during or after the operation
- damage to other organs
- infection
- thrombosis (blood clots)
- death

Let's deal with the most difficult risk first: the overall risk of maternal death from Cesarean section is 20 in 100,000 operations, or 0.0002 percent. Women do die in Cesarean surgery, but rarely. A death in Cesarean surgery may be caused by the medical condition that made the surgery necessary, eclampsia, reaction to anesthetic, bleeding disorders, or postoperative complications. Cesarean surgery very seldom causes the baby to die. Instead, the condition that made surgery necessary in the first place is the most common cause of infant death during C-section.

We discussed the risks of anesthesia in chapter 3, so we won't go over them again here.

Bleeding

Cassie went into labor with her first pregnancy one week past her due date and arrived in the labor ward with contractions five minutes apart. Her first exam showed that she was three centimeters dilated, which is normal. Almost immediately after she was settled into her bed, her water broke. But her doctor was concerned that, along with amniotic fluid, there was bright red blood. When the bleeding stopped, everyone breathed a sigh of relief and hoped there would be no further cause for alarm. Within 10 minutes, however, there was another gush of bright red blood, this time accompanied by meconium, the greenish black fetal feces that signals fetal distress. The monitor showed some flattening of the baby's heartbeat. Cassie's doctor recommended urgent C-section.

By the time Cassie reached the OR, minutes later, the baby's heart rate had slowed to 70. Cassie had an epidural in place, but she was not getting adequate pain relief, so the anesthesiologist put her under general anesthesia. Time was of the essence. Her daughter's first Apgar score was on the low side, but Hilda quickly perked up under the expert ministrations of her attending pediatrician. (See appendix B for Apgar rating.)

The cause of Cassie's bleeding was a partially separated placenta. Cassie also bled more than usual during the surgery, and her hemoglobin dropped down to 7 (in women, normal hemoglobin is greater than 12.5). Cassie needed a transfusion of two units of blood. Before the end of a week, though, Cassie and Hilda were settled in at home.

Some bleeding is an inevitable part of having a C-section. After the incision is made into the uterus and before the baby is taken out of the uterus, the bleeding is heavy from the raw, cut edges of the wound. Soon after the baby is delivered, however, the mother is given a medication that helps her uterus to contract down and helps close off the bleeding vessels, slowing the bleeding. At the same time, the surgeon stitches the wound closed, which stops the bleeding.

There is some risk that the surgical cut into the uterus will extend into the larger blood vessels that supply the placenta or into a branch of the main artery to the uterus. Any cutting of these blood-carrying vessels is, of course, unintentional. In this situation, the surgeon acts quickly to stop this bleeding by clamping or stitching closed the bleeding blood vessels. During training, the surgeon was given extensive practice in closing off blood vessels, and the necessary tools are always on hand during any operation. Rarely, a transfusion will be needed: about one in 50 of the women who bleed because of cut vessels will need a transfusion. The possibility of the need for transfusion is increased in women who have already had significant blood loss, for example, from placenta previa. In fact, they may need transfusion for that reason alone.

Some women get a nasty surprise with vaginal bleeding after surgery, while they are recovering. This is slightly more common in women who have had general anesthesia than in women who have had spinal or epidural anesthesia because of the muscle relaxant drugs used in general anesthesia. These drugs can prevent the uterine muscle from contracting as firmly as needed; when the uterus does not contract properly, drugs called *oxytocics* are administered to cause the uterus to contract. A "lazy" uterus can occur after any type of childbirth, including vaginal, and is treated the same way whenever it occurs.

A slipped stitch is another possible reason for bleeding. A slipped stitch is a stitch that has slipped off the blood vessel it was closing. Often the bleeding settles down after a dose of medication to make the uterus contract, but sometimes a transfusion or a trip back to the operating room to reopen the incision, find the bleeder, and reclose it may be necessary. The most accurate figure we've found for the risk of bleeding from a slipped stitch in C-section is about one in one thousand C-sections, or 0.001 percent.

These days many women are more afraid of transfusion than of blood loss. This is not justified because U.S. blood supplies are very carefully screened and are very safe. Sometimes, rather than donated blood, a blood substitute is used when fluid replacement is necessary, especially for women who have a religious objection to blood transfusion. There is always a possibility of an adverse reaction to blood transfusion, almost an allergic reaction that occurs at the time of transfusion. Transfusions are carefully monitored, with Benadryl at hand in case of a reaction. Women tolerate lower hemoglobins than we previously thought; thus, rather than giving the mother a blood transfusion, we might help her replenish her iron supplies after birth by prescribing iron-rich foods and iron supplements. (See appendix D for iron-rich foods.)

The decision about how to compensate for substantial blood loss must be made on an individual basis. A woman having an elective

Cesarean can discuss her preferences with her doctor beforehand. Most doctors will try to go along with the patient's wishes, but the doctor must ultimately do what is best for the patient's health, unless the patient has written instructions against transfusion (as Jehovah's Witnesses do, for example). A doctor performing an emergency C-section will use his or her best judgment to protect the patient's health. Going home anemic will lengthen a mother's recovery time. She will be more tired and will need to honor her need for rest.

The topic of transfusion raises the topic of *autologous blood banking,* which means giving and storing your own blood in case blood is needed during the surgery. It is not unusual for blood to be taken and stored when someone is planning elective surgery in which a transfusion may be needed. This is not a common practice for the prospect of C-section, however, in part because the hemodynamics of pregnancy are different from the hemodynamics of nonpregnancy. Pregnancy is not a good time to be giving blood, even if it is for your own possible future use. All of your blood is needed for the development of the baby. (*Hemodynamics* is the movement of blood and the forces involved in the movement of blood.)

Damage to Other Organs
DAMAGE TO THE BLADDER

Pregnancy makes nearly every woman very aware of the relationship between her enlarging uterus and her bladder. In labor or at term, the baby's head (or other presenting part) is located right up against the bladder (separated by the uterine wall, of course). Making the "smiley face" incision of C-section, the surgeon needs to be exquisitely careful to avoid cutting or nicking the bladder. The insertion of that undignified and uncomfortable catheter helps keep the bladder empty, small, and out of the way of the incision. Dissection into the abdomen proceeds very carefully, layer by layer, until the bladder is seen and can be held out of harm's way. This care is repeated during the stitching. Even with these precautions, however, every obstetrician who has performed many Cesareans will admit that he or she has punctured a woman's bladder from time to time. Thank goodness it is a very forgiving organ!

Paolina was having her third C-section. Unfortunately, scar tissue from her previous Cesarean sections made her bladder tightly adhere to the front wall of her uterus. Paolina's third child, Chiara, weighed close to 10 pounds at birth. In the process of taking Chiara out of the womb, the doctor accidentally tore Paolina's bladder. After sewing Paolina's uterus closed, her obstetrician repaired her bladder, stitching together the torn edges, much as you'd repair a torn gown. To allow the bladder to rest and heal, Paolina had to wear a catheter for 10 days. This was a bit awkward, but she was fitted up with a bag taped to her thigh, and no one was the wiser. As she said, "It certainly wasn't as though I was going out dancing in that week. I tried to think of it as saving me having to get up to pee at night." After the catheter was removed, Paolina's "water works" were as good as new. Two years later, she had a fourth and last C-section with no complications, bladder or otherwise.

Previous surgeries, whether C-sections or other types of operation, may cause scar adhesions to form between the bladder and the uterus, making it more difficult to separate the two organs. This is what happened with Paolina. A big baby may also make it necessary to extend the uterine incision. Both of these situations increase the possibility of tearing the bladder. A large study indicated that injury was sustained by the bladder in one in six hundred C-sections (less than 0.002%); less often, the ureters were injured. Most injuries in this study occurred in repeat or complicated C-sections.

Another infrequent problem after C-section is not being able to urinate once the catheter is removed. There are many tips to help you to relax and let it go, such as running water, sitting in a warm bath, and directing the shower spray on your lower abdomen. Inability to void is a side effect of the surgery plus the anesthetic and is more apt to happen if you have a C-section after many hours of labor. Sometimes the catheter has to go back in for a few days.

There is no cause for worry because the problem will resolve and you *will* be able to urinate.

DAMAGE TO THE BOWEL OR RECTUM

Damage to the bowel or rectum is much less common than damage to the bladder because the bowel and rectum are not within the field of surgery. When damage does occur, it is almost always associated with some previous surgery or some unusual complication, such as the need for a Cesarean hysterectomy (see below).

The bowel can be just as sluggish as the bladder in resuming normal function, however. Again, this is more common in women who labored long or who had extensive previous abdominal surgery. Being a little sluggish is normal, but once in a blue moon, the bowel can become completely still for a time. Called *paralytic ileus,* this condition occurs in about one of each five hundred C-sections (0.002%). We treat it by keeping the bowel empty. IV fluids are necessary because the patient can have nothing by mouth. To avoid paralytic ileus, we allow only sips of liquids and then small amounts of soft foods in the first 24 hours, as we saw in Emily's story.

Infection

Two types of infection are commonly associated with C-sections: bladder infection and infection in the surgical wound and uterus. There are risks of infection in vaginal delivery, as well. In vaginal delivery, minor tears in the cervix and vagina are not unusual; because the opening of the vagina and the entrance to the urethra are located close to the rectum, contamination with fecal bacteria may cause vaginal or bladder infection. Also, once the placenta is delivered, a raw, open area exists where the placenta was previously located, and infections sometimes develop in this area (infection in this area led to many deaths before the age of antibiotics).

As we've noted, the bladder lies very close to the uterus and must be catheterized before C-section. Catheterization can introduce bacteria, even though every effort is made to follow procedures that minimize the risk of infection. Bladder infections are easily treated, partly because doctors catch them early (because doctors have a high level of suspicion that they might occur) and also because bladder infections respond well to antibiotics. When an infection is suspected, a sample of urine is taken and cultured to see whether bacteria grow, but commonly, antibiotics are begun before we have the culture results.

These days, most doctors administer a prophylactic, broad-spectrum antibiotic when performing a C-section. In many uncomplicated cases, this is a single dose. If there are other indications, such as a fever in labor, repeated vaginal exams in labor, a long time since rupture of membranes (water breaking), or vaginal group B strep infection, antibiotics are used for a longer time. Properly conducted trials have confirmed that this regimen is effective in preventing infection in the uterus or in the external wound.

Deep Vein Thrombosis and Pulmonary Embolism

During labor, blood may pool and stagnate in the veins of the legs and pelvis. This is most likely to happen if the woman has been confined to her labor bed with an epidural in place. Whenever a person does not move his or her legs for a prolonged period, clots are more likely to form in the veins. A clot such as this (called *deep vein thrombosis*) may break off, in whole or in part, and travel through the veins to the lungs (a *pulmonary embolism*), blocking the blood vessels there and causing extreme breathing difficulties and even sudden death. Compounding the nightmare, these conditions are even more likely to occur in pregnancy because two hormones necessary to sustain a pregnancy increase the risk of thrombosis. The hormone *estrogen* makes the blood thicker and stickier, and the hormone *progesterone* makes the smooth muscle in the walls of veins relax.

The good news is that we can take very effective steps to prevent these conditions. Many devices are used, but you will be most aware of your TED stockings: ugly white elastic stockings, with a hole for your toes. You will be encouraged to keep wearing them postop, at least until you go home. They make no fashion statement and they are the very devil to get on, but they are much better than blood clots.

Other approaches include calf compressors, large air bags that are strapped to your legs and that inflate and deflate intermittently to pump the blood through your leg veins and back to your heart. Calf stimulators are also used. They send electrical messages to your leg muscles, causing them to contract and pump the blood back to your heart. You may be unaware of these devices because they are used during your operation, and you are either asleep or have your mind on other matters—such as seeing your baby. If you are at very high risk of developing deep vein thrombosis, a blood thinner called *heparin* may be started postop. This is used with great caution because it acts to decrease the clotting activity in the blood; therefore, its obvious side effect is bleeding, which, of course, is to be avoided. Use of heparin requires a careful weighing of the risks and benefits.

Cesarean Hysterectomy

During a C-section life-threatening problems do, rarely, occur and make it necessary to perform a hysterectomy. Nearly always the problem is severe hemorrhaging, and nearly always the hemorrhaging is caused by placenta previa, often along with other risk factors. When you sign your consent form for your C-section, you will note that hysterectomy is mentioned as a possible consequence of the C-section, but hysterectomy during C-section is as rare as hen's teeth in all but the circumstances just mentioned. In such a procedure, all or part of the uterus is removed, usually just enough to stop the bleeding. The ovaries are not removed.

In this chapter we have discussed the risks you should be aware of, not only if you contemplate an elective C-section but also if you plan a vaginal delivery, just in case a Cesarean should end up being necessary. We hope we have made it clear that most of these problems can be anticipated and prevented or treated if they occur. We mentioned earlier that the maternal death rate with C-section is 20 in 100,000; we want to emphasize that these deaths are associated with the complications of C-section and rarely occur with uncomplicated procedures. It is also only fair to point out that there are risks with vaginal delivery as well; pelvic floor repair is uncommon in women who have had Cesareans, for example, and C-section in itself poses fewer risks to the baby than vaginal delivery does.

PART II

ॐ ॐ ॐ

WHAT'S NEXT? AFTER A CESAREAN SECTION

CHAPTER 7

ॐ ॐ ॐ

Going Home
You and Your Family

Going home with a new baby and a fresh scar on your belly can be a daunting prospect. You suddenly feel all the vulnerabilities that every new mother feels: Can I be the perfect mother this little guy deserves? How can I protect my baby so nothing bad happens to her? But, in addition to these normal vulnerabilities, if you have had a C-section you will also have some pain, you will be tired, and your body will have a fair amount of healing to do. Your body must recover from major surgery and possibly from general anesthesia, as well. If you are returning home to problems, such as money or family worries, or if you have concerns about your personal relationships or your job, the days and weeks ahead of you will be even more challenging.

Unless you live just around the corner from the hospital, even the trip home will be surprisingly tiring. You can expect to feel tired, especially in the first few days home. This is normal. Our advice is to pamper yourself. Whenever you feel like it, if you can, *go to bed and take a nap*—no matter what time of day or how long the line of people wanting to visit or how high the stack of tasks waiting to be tackled. Needless to say, at least during the first week home from the hospital, you will need some help. Your family and friends will almost certainly be glad to pitch in to care for you, your baby, and your other children. Take the support that's offered! You will recover more quickly if you don't overdo things. Also, this is one of those times to ask for help if you need help. People may not think to offer, but they will be pleased to be asked. You will be able to repay their generosity in the future.

A *doula* may be just what you need. A doula is a person who takes care of you so you can take care of your baby. Any of the caring people in your life can be your doula, or you may be able to hire a professional doula. Your need for the services of a doula depends upon the number of children you have at home, including the new baby. For a little while, all you'll be able to handle is eating, sleeping, bathing, breast-feeding, and giving loving attention to your children. Your doula will take care of everything else!

There are some practical concerns that may catch you by surprise—for example, the first time you're sitting in a chair with the baby and you need to go to the toilet and there's no one to help you get up! For at least the first couple of weeks after the baby is born, you will not be able to use your stomach muscles to get up from a chair—you will need your hands to push off. When you have the baby in your arms, your doula or someone else needs to take the baby from you so you can get up. Our advice is to plan ahead!

Holding the baby to breast-feed may be challenging at first, too. In the hospital, you probably mastered the technique of putting a folded blanket or pillow on your lap to hold the weight of the baby. At home, your partner, your doula, or someone else will need to help you by bringing the baby to you and helping to settle the baby comfortably against you. You won't have to use your muscles very much, and you can avoid some discomfort and strain. After the baby nurses, your helper can burp the baby and perhaps settle him or her down for a nap. Drinking lots of fluid while you are nursing helps your milk supply and your recovery.

The warmth of a shower against your full breasts and the healing scar on your belly feels heavenly. After the shower, you may want to rub vitamin E oil or cocoa butter on your scar to keep it lubricated and decrease itching. The stubble of shaved hair on your pubis can be an itchy misery, too; keep it soft with lotion—or continue to shave and deal with the hair growing in later. A folded silk scarf nestled in your undies may also soften the itch until you are fully healed.

Every young mother is advised to nap when the baby naps, and too few of us heed this advice. Believe us, this is one of the most sensible things you can do, especially if you have other young children. Develop blinders for "the things that should get done." Remember that an inch of dust is just as easy to remove as an infinitesimal speck of it—and infinitely more gratifying! This time in your life is about "quality survival," not about the ideal.

You will find that vacuuming, mopping, sweeping, and shoveling are fatiguing out of all proportion to their difficulty or the time they take. There is something about that combination of swiveling at the hip and using the arms that is very difficult after abdominal surgery. Let someone else do these tasks until you are at least two months postop. (You are medically capable earlier, but never mind that.)

Exercise

As soon as your doctor gives you the OK, you should begin doing exercises to tone up those poor abused belly muscles. After all they've been through, their natural tendency now is to sag. Saggy abdominal muscles contribute to backaches, and strong abdominal muscles help prevent backache. Appearance and self-image aside, avoiding backache is a good reason to begin exercising after you are healed.

Start your exercise program slowly, with just a couple of minutes at first. Your weakened muscles are more likely to cramp and strain than are muscles that haven't been stretched, so take it gently. As your muscle strength returns, increase your exercise time to 15 minutes daily.

It's not likely that you will be leaving home regularly for exercise or any other reason at this stage, so we have in mind a home program, not one that requires you to go anywhere. On the other hand, swimming is great fun and good exercise, so if you have access to water and your doctor has given you the OK, then take the plunge! Gentle yoga is another excellent postdelivery possibility. Be careful just now of any sports that may exhaust you, however—

like tennis, squash, handball, and contact sports. They can come later.

We offer the five exercises below as a simple approach to toning your muscles. Wear loose, comfortable clothing. You may do the exercises on the floor, on carpeting, or on an exercise mat. Many people inadvertently hold their breath while exercising! Don't do that—be sure to breathe in and out as you go.

1. *Knee to shoulder.* Lie on your back with your knees bent and your feet flat on the floor. Cup your hands around one knee and draw that leg up to your chest. Hold it in place while you breathe in and out deeply four times. Repeat about five times with each leg.

2. *Cat stretch.* Get up on your hands and knees on the floor. Align your body parallel with the floor, and then arch your back like a Halloween cat. Hold this position and breathe in and out twice. Then lower your back to the starting position and repeat. If you have other children, they may get in the act with you. Children love this stretch. Repeat about five times.

3. *Sit-up.* Lie on your back with your knees bent and your feet flat on the floor. Now, reach up with your hands for your knees. This should raise your shoulders off the floor, and you should feel the pull in your belly. Hold yourself in this position for one deep breath and then curl back down. Repeat five times.

4. *Pelvic tilt.* Lie on your back with your knees bent and your feet flat on the floor. Tighten your buttocks and roll your pelvis so that the small of your back is touching the floor. Hold this position for three deep breaths and then return to your starting position. Repeat five times.

5. *Leg lift.* Lie on your stomach and raise your left leg straight up behind you as far as you can without raising your hips from the floor. Lower your left leg and then raise your right leg. Hold each leg up as long as you can. Don't forget to breathe. Repeat each leg lift five times.

These five exercises may seem almost too simple, but if you are faithful with them, they will return the muscle tone to your abdomen and help you feel fit and trim. *And* you can do them without ever having your children out of sight. How can you lose?

Nutrition

A common concern of women who've just delivered is that they will have to diet very strictly to lose the weight they gained. What they need to consider at this time, however, is the *quality* of what they eat, not how little they can get by with. A woman who has just delivered a baby needs adequate nutrients to feel well—even more so if she is breast-feeding. A nursing mother's body will make sure that her milk is nutritious for the baby, even if this nutrition is gained at the expense of the mother's own health. Eat!

Some of us forget to eat when we are busy or stressed. And some of us fix healthy meals for our children and eat only what the children leave behind. But your child's mother needs to be well fed, too! You can give your child a better routine if you have a routine for yourself. Eating doesn't have to be a five-course meal, but it should be more than a candy bar and soda or coffee and a doughnut or tea and cookies. Many such snack foods provide empty calories and leave you tired and irritable and with your extra weight still hanging about.

Eat as much protein and vegetables and fruits as you need to satisfy your hunger. Include oils in your diet. Avoid processed foods, including many kinds of bread and cereal; get your carbohydrates instead from vegetables, fruits, and whole grains. By following this approach to nutrition, especially if you are breast-feeding, you will lose the weight you have gained. Sound too simple? Not really, because the foods commonly eaten in excess are processed carbohydrates and foods that are combinations of processed carbohydrate and fat. Chips, for example. And doughnuts. No patient of ours has ever reported insatiable cravings for bell peppers or fish or olive oil. We have found that the "carb cravings" just go away when a person gives the body enough of these other foods. Try it. You, too, may find that you feel more satisfied and less hungry.

Fish is a source of protein and good fatty acids, but we must issue a caution about some fish that, in our times, unfortunately, are contaminated by environmental toxins such as PCBs, PBBs, and mercury. While pregnant or breast-feeding, enjoy cod, pollock, and haddock often, and eat salmon, flounder, and sole no more than once a week. Avoid tuna, bluefish, catfish, striped bass, shark, and swordfish, however, as they are too likely to contain high levels of contaminants. Check with your state health department to find out about locally caught fish. Also, skip the sushi bar while you are pregnant: raw fish may have bacterial contaminants.

It is well known that avoiding alcohol during your first three months of pregnancy is very important because alcohol is damaging to the fetus. After the first trimester of pregnancy, the occasional glass of wine or beer is not disastrous, but drinking on a regular basis is still to be avoided. What about alcohol after childbirth? The authors were raised in Ireland with the traditional idea of a glass of stout daily for each nursing mother and, over the years, have found it not a bad idea. Stout relaxes you and does have good food value. It is not of such great value that you should try to develop a taste for stout if you don't like it, however. Small amounts of most other alcoholic drinks may be relaxing, but they contribute empty calories. Of course, consume all alcohol in moderation. You would not want to be robbed of awareness during the few free moments you have in a day, whether you are nursing or not.

Sex

There are times in every woman's life when sex is very low on the list of priorities, and the postpartum period is commonly one of them. Don't worry—interest in sexual activity returns. You are advised not to have intercourse for about six weeks after a Cesarean section, in any case, because of some danger of infection.

Most women get their doctor's green light to resume sexual relations at their six-week checkup. But not every woman is ready to feel good about sex at six weeks postop. Some women are still feeling fatigued and overwhelmed by the whole experience and are happy just to get through each day, hitting the bed with a prayer that the baby will sleep at least three hours. Some women experience vaginal dryness associated with the hormonal changes of delivery and breast-feeding, and this can make sexual relations physically uncomfortable. The good news is that, since you haven't had an episiotomy, you won't be sore in the area around the opening to the vagina. Studies have shown that, in the first six months after their first vaginal delivery, approximately 85 percent of women have some discomfort in this area. For a woman who has a C-section, her incision may trouble her for the first six weeks but generally not after that.

Once your doctor says it's OK, if you *are* interested in sex, you may appreciate a few hints to make sex more comfortable and enjoyable. For example, choose positions that limit penetration, such as the spooning position. A vaginal lubricant such as Replens or KY jelly will help if you are dry; apply it liberally. Try to plan time for sex when you are not tired; what you lose in spontaneity you will make up for in energy.

Finally, be sure you feel secure in your choice of birth control; nothing can dampen interest like the fear of pregnancy, especially soon after the birth of a child. (See chap. 9 for a discussion of different birth control methods.)

We have found that a woman's interest in sex returns more readily when she is well nourished and well rested. For this reason and so many others, she must not neglect taking care of herself. Her family will be happier and will function better if she is in good health, physically and emotionally.

You may at times feel as if sex is just another obligation to one of your loved ones. All of us have probably felt this at one time or other. In our view, it is OK to have sex for the love of your partner and not because of any desire or need of your own. This is part of a contract of love and is not self-disrespectful. It is part of what holds a relationship together. Having sex if it feels wrong to you is not the same thing at all, however; this *is* disrespectful of yourself.

Talk your feelings over with your partner, and work through this time together. It may be that hugs and kisses will get you through. We all need plenty of support and affection, and hugs are very powerful medicine. Sometimes, we just need to be held.

CHAPTER 8

⨳ ⨳ ⨳

Postpartum Depression

In this chapter we provide information to help new mothers understand and cope with depression after delivery. You may still be coping with these feelings long after delivery, or you may simply want to have a better understanding of an experience that is now part of your past. Either way, we hope this chapter is helpful; we also point the way to other sources of help and encourage you to turn to these sources if you need to.

Lucy, a young mother who had suffered a rupture of the uterus during a trial of labor, was very depressed after the loss of her baby. Within hours she had gone from being a happy, expectant mother to being a grieving mother who had lost her baby and the possibility of a future pregnancy. She was also suffering from anemia caused by the blood loss she had sustained. Deadened to all feeling, she was certain her life would never get any better. Fortunately, she had a gifted psychologist and a husband who is a candidate for sainthood. Toby took over all care of their living child, Edith, who was two years old at the time, and did his own mourning in private. All of his energies were directed toward helping to heal his family and go on.

Jan's mild depression after her C-section delivery was a product of her hormonal vulnerability after pregnancy and her very real disappointment and feelings of failure that she had not been able to birth her baby "naturally." Her disappointment eased with time and as she talked with her doctor and her family and friends about what had happened. She also formed a support group with a few other "Cesarean moms," just to talk and share experiences. Jan came to understand that she had done the best thing possible for her baby.

Casey was 19 years old when Ryan was born after a brutal 28-hour labor. Ryan weighed 10 pounds, 4 ounces, and Casey is only five feet tall and normally weighs about 105 pounds soaking wet. Her vagina was badly torn and, from that day on, her back always hurt and intercourse hurt. When Casey became pregnant with her second child, she begged her obstetrician from the very beginning to do a C-section. "No, no, you're a strong young woman and you've already shown that you can deliver a large baby vaginally," was the reply.

As the due date approached, Casey became more and more nervous, and she cried again as she begged for a Cesarean. Again, her doctor answered: "You just have to trust me. I know what is best for you and your baby, and you don't want a big scar on your belly. Your husband wouldn't like that, now would he?" Finally, after another long labor and another 10-pound baby, Casey finished her family.

Casey was so badly injured during her deliveries that now, in her very early thirties, she needs a pelvic floor repair operation. Having sex is excruciatingly painful. But that's not why we're telling her story now. We're telling her story because, after her second birth, Casey slumped into a severe depression, taking no joy in life and feeling gloomy about the future. She was on antidepressant medication for many months and couldn't breast-feed Colin, her second son.

Casey came to understand, through months of therapy with a good psychiatrist, that in addition to the physical trauma she suffers, she feels abused because she was denied the right to make decisions about her own body. Part of her healing process was writing a letter to the obstetrician who treated her in what she considered an inhumane way. She told him exactly how she felt and said that, although nothing could change how things turned out for her, she did expect an apology.

Lucy, Jan, and Casey all had postpartum depression. Lucy's depression left her unable to carry on the activities of daily life. Jan felt sad and disappointed. Casey was desperately unhappy and angry, as well. These are just some of the faces of depression, which shows up in different ways in different people. When depression is recognized and properly treated, people with depression have a much better chance of recovering quickly and completely. Jan recovered with time and informal support. Both Lucy and Casey benefited from "talking therapy" with a professional counselor, and Casey was helped by medications.

One study showed that 50–80 percent of women experience "the blues" after giving birth. Not *true* depression, but instead a heightened emotionality, the blues reach a peak in the first week after delivery and usually even out by the end of the second postpartum week. The shifts of hormones after delivery undoubtedly have much to do with these sad feelings, but there is also the letdown after nine months of waiting and preparing for the event that is now past, leaving us with permanently changed lives. Some women have very real practical problems to deal with now—such as being a single mother or having to return immediately to work because of economic necessity. Being the mother of a newborn often is not easy. As a rule, true depression hits a bit later than "the blues," although, of course, one may slide into the other. Also, postpartum depression tends to last longer than the baby blues—it may persist for a year or more.

How common is postpartum or postnatal depression? True postpartum depression occurs in 10–50 percent of mothers, depending upon which study you consult. Studies in women in war-torn Lebanon found an incidence of postpartum depression close to 50 percent, but we have to think that a good part of this was situational; it seems natural that women who have a new baby to raise in a dangerous setting like war will feel afraid and anxious and depressed.

How can we define postpartum depression? We have to rely on symptoms of thinking and feeling much more than on bodily symptoms like fatigue and sleep disturbance because these physical symptoms are common in new mothers. The thinking and feeling symptoms include blaming yourself for lots of things, losing all sense of humor, feeling sad and unhappy most of the time, not looking forward to anything pleasurable, crying, and, possibly, having thoughts of harming yourself. A very small percentage of mothers (2 in 1,000, or 0.002 percent) will have a very extreme form of depression and may have hallucinations or paranoid delusions; such women may be at real danger of harming themselves or their babies.

There may be warning signs of impending postpartum depression. It occurs more often in women who are depressed during pregnancy, for example, although it can also affect women who have never suffered depression. Postpartum depression is more common after a failed trial of labor because the woman's expectations for vaginal birth may have been unrealistically high. Postpartum depression may also be more common in older mothers. It is more likely to recur after subsequent pregnancies if it had occurred in one pregnancy. We know one woman who suffered from depression after the birth of both of her first two children and had to be hospitalized after her third child was born; she had become fixated on the idea that she should kill her baby because there was no way she could be a good mother. She had slipped into postpartum psychosis, and the danger to her baby was real, as we recently saw in the media reports about the poor woman in Texas who drowned her five children.

Other risk factors for postpartum depression are

- a family history of depression, especially a prior personal episode
- a poor relationship with one's partner, especially if abuse is involved
- isolation from friends and family
- lack of help with childcare
- lack of social supports
- substance abuse
- anxiety disorder

Having listed these risk factors, we must emphasize that *every* woman is at risk of postpartum depression. This disorder transcends cultures and socioeconomic classes.

Treatment may be as simple as providing supportive, loving care and temporarily shifting responsibilities off the new mother, or it may involve medication or hospitalization. Counseling is provided by a variety of professionals, including clergy, psychologists, psychiatrists, and social workers. Only medical doctors (M.D.s) such as family doctors, internists, or psychiatrists can prescribe medications. The newer antidepressants have been an enormous help for many women. Recently, some researchers have found that small doses of estrogen may be helpful in treating postpartum depression. For severe or ongoing depression, it's often recommended that the person consult a psychiatrist, who has experience with different antidepressants and other drugs for mood disorders. The person may still consult a psychologist, social worker, or clergy for talking therapy and counseling.

Postpartum depression may cause difficulties with breast-feeding, such as difficulty positioning the baby (because of anxiety), decreased milk supply, and problems with letdown of milk. A woman who wants to breast-feed her newborn may feel even sadder if she is unable to nurse successfully. If a woman needs antidepressant medication, her doctor will probably choose one of the older tricyclic antidepressants at the lowest effective dose because it is safer for the baby.

If you feel blue or sad or if you experience depression after your baby is born, don't suffer in silence or feel ashamed. Fully 25 percent of affected women will still be depressed a year after delivery if they are not treated. Getting treatment means there is less of a chance that the quality will be robbed from your life and your children's lives. Tell your doctor about your feelings and get help. Doing so is important for you and your family.

CHAPTER 9

కౌ కౌ కౌ

Contraception

You are settled back in at home. Your doctor has told you that your recovery is complete and you can resume sexual relations. The birth of this baby may herald the completion of family goals, or it may bracket a time to regain energy and strength and to enjoy this baby before becoming pregnant again. But even if you want a large family, it's not likely that you will want to become pregnant again right away. And if you have had a Cesarean section, you should wait at least three months to let your scar heal before you become pregnant again.

Breast-feeding interferes with fertility to some extent, although breast-feeding is not a foolproof method of birth control. If you are not breast-feeding, your periods are likely to return about six weeks after delivery, and you should assume that you are then able to conceive.

A natural curb on fertility at this time is a decrease in libido. Most women have very little interest in sex right now. *This is normal.* Your libido will return, but for the time being your body is dealing with survival: eating, sleeping, and feeding the baby are your body's priorities—sexuality just doesn't rank high. It's helpful if your partner understands that lack of libido is a normal physiological response to childbirth and that your decreased interest in sex has nothing to do with your feelings for him. Most couples don't resume intercourse until six to eight weeks after the delivery, and some wait even longer.

But abstinence generally is not a long-term solution to preventing pregnancy, and avoiding intercourse because you are afraid of getting pregnant is not good for your relationship in the long run. What are you going to do about birth control, then? There are many ways to prevent conception besides abstinence. In this chapter we discuss the pros and cons of these various methods of contraception (see p. 110 for a table summarizing these methods).

Breast-feeding

First let's talk about breast-feeding, which for thousands of years has been known to interfere with conception. It is true that, if you are fully breast-feeding, you are less likely to become pregnant. A fully breast-feeding woman has a less than 2 percent chance of becoming pregnant in the first six months of full breast-feeding because the low levels of some hormones during breast-feeding prevent ovulation. Population studies also make it clear that breast-feeding accounts for an average of two years between pregnancies. Breast-feeding in conjunction with properly used condoms, a diaphragm, or another method of birth control is very effective.

Data about breast-feeding and pregnancy are based on a large population of women, *some* of whom *did* get pregnant while breast-feeding. If you do not wish to become pregnant, do not rely exclusively on breast-feeding as a birth control method.

You notice that we use the term *fully breast-feeding*. If you are giving supplemental foods or partially weaning, the birth control protection of breast-feeding will not be as effective as it is when the breast is the baby's sole source of nutrition. The menstrual cycles of women who supplement the breast and of women who are well nourished return much quicker than those of women who breast-feed exclusively or who have marginalized nutrition. Michele has a fond memory of going to an all-you-can-eat buffet when her baby was about six months old: "I went back and filled my plate about four times. Finally, I stopped out of embarrassment when I realized that I was the cause of much amusement for the people sitting near us."

If you are breast-feeding, you may note vaginal dryness that causes pain with intercourse. This dryness occurs because the estrogen levels have dropped off due to breast-feeding. The dryness is temporary and can be counteracted with over-the-counter lubricants such as Replens and KY jelly or with prescription vaginal estrogen, which is available in the form of creams, tablets, or suppositories. These vaginal estrogens are safe because very little of the estrogen is systemically absorbed (absorbed by the bloodstream and tissues).

Natural Family Planning

Natural family planning is any method of contraception that involves determining when you are fertile and then abstaining from intercourse during this time. All methods of natural family planning rely on the woman being very familiar with her menstrual cycle and being aware of the signs of her fertile time.

To use natural family planning, a woman must be able to predict when she is going to ovulate. There are several ways of doing this.

1. Some women designate days 9 through 17 of their cycle, beginning with the first day of the menstrual period as day 1, as the "unsafe days." This is a chancy approach, unless you have an extremely predictable 28-day cycle. This is often called the *rhythm method*.

2. Some women take their temperature before they get out of bed in the morning. This temperature is the *basal body temperature*. Just after ovulation, your basal temperature goes up a little and it stays slightly elevated for two or three days. Because the elevation is only a part of a degree, you need a thermometer marked off in tenths of a degree, designed for family-planning purposes.

3. Noting changes in your cervical mucus is called the *Billings method*. If you reach a finger into your vagina, you feel a knob similar to the end of your nose. This is your cervix. It has a small opening covered with mucus. During most of the month, this mucus is thick and sticky. When you ovulate, the mucus becomes thin and runny, like egg white. Also like egg

white, it can stretch out like a thread. Unfortunately, sometimes things such as sexual excitement can change the quality of the cervical mucus and lead to error. The *symptothermal method* combines basal body temperature and tests of cervical mucus.

4. Some women experience a pain at the time of ovulation. This pain may be sharp or dull and may last from a few minutes to a few hours. It usually occurs on just one side. Also, some women may have slight spotting of blood at this time. These are useful signs for the woman wanting to use natural family planning.

Once you have determined when you ovulate, you and your partner must agree to abstain from intercourse altogether or use a barrier method during this time. Most women are fertile for about three days after ovulation. Keep in mind that while you are breast-feeding you may not have a period for about six months and that you will ovulate about two weeks before that period, so natural family methods are unreliable during breast-feeding.

Natural family planning requires daily vigilance and a cooperative partner. Although theoretically this is a very good method, in practice the rate of pregnancy for women using natural family planning is 18–25 percent, depending on how carefully the method is followed. Therefore, the risk of pregnancy must be an acceptable risk.

Barrier Methods

When we talk of barrier methods, we mean literally a barrier between the sperm and the cervix. Barrier methods, including condoms, diaphragms, sponges, and caps, haven't changed much over the past century, although the female condom is a new development. Used in conjunction with breast-feeding, barrier methods have a low failure rate. On their own, the failure rate is about 12–18 percent for the male condom and 2–20 percent for the diaphragm.

For maximum protection, all barrier methods need to be used with *every* act of intercourse, and used properly. Too often the failure of barrier methods is due to leaving the barrier in the drawer or being careless in putting it on or in properly.

For greatest effectiveness, the male condom must cover the entire shaft of the penis, it must be put on before any penetration takes place, and a space must be left at the end of the condom so the semen can pool there and not overflow at the top. Female condoms are also available, but thus far they haven't been greeted with much enthusiasm. Perhaps they will be improved and will be used by more women in the future. If you use a diaphragm or cap for contraception, get your diaphragm or cap refitted after every pregnancy. Your body changes with pregnancy and childbirth, and you may need a different size now. Your doctor can check your size at your six-week checkup.

Some women liked the Today sponge, which is not currently available—although an updated version of the sponge will be available soon. To use the sponge, you moisten it and insert it into your vagina. The only problem with the sponge, aside from the risk of unplanned pregnancy ("failures"), is a potential hypersensitivity reaction to the spermicide in the sponge. Stop using the sponge if you have a reaction. When it is again available, you will be able to purchase the sponge without a prescription, over the counter. It has about a 15 percent failure rate.

The Pill

Ideally you should wait until your six-week checkup and the return of your period before starting the pill, to allow your body to resume normal cycling. If you have intercourse before this, you should use a barrier method. Some doctors prefer to start their patients on the pill as soon as they leave the hospital, fearing that otherwise they will become pregnant. No one knows better than you whether you actually *will* use the barrier methods or whether you are apt "to take your chances." Be realistic. This is life, not a quiz with right and wrong answers.

If you are going to "go on the pill," you should use a barrier method in addition until you have taken the pill for at least seven days, because there is a possibility that you ovulated before the pill took effect, and you may need the additional protection. The pill has a failure rate of less than 1 percent.

Birth-control pills containing estrogen can interfere with the hormonal control that regulates breast-feeding. Taking birth-control pills can reduce or even stop milk production. If you are breast-feeding, you do not want to take pills containing estrogen. You can use the progesterone-only pill, or "mini-pill," however, taking this pill with the assurance that it does provide you with good protection. You should not start taking this pill immediately after giving birth because your progesterone levels are still very high then, and they need to fall to normal postpartum levels. Usually this happens by the third or fourth day after delivery.

The progesterone-only pill is very reliable, with a pregnancy rate of less than 1 percent. Initially you may notice some bleeding and spotting, but this will settle down, and then you may go without periods for a long time. This is a normal effect of this type of pill and is no cause for worry.

If you are not breast-feeding, you may use any of the combination-type pills as long as you have no medical contraindication, such as high blood pressure, a history of blood clots, or severe migraines. You and your doctor should thoroughly discuss your health and the pros and cons of the birth-control pill before you begin taking pills. The pregnancy rate with these pills, when taken conscientiously, is less than 1 percent.

IUDs

IUDs (intrauterine devices) used to be far more popular and more widely available than they are today. They were also much less expensive. The cost of IUDs was driven up and the availability was decreased after lawsuits over the Dalkon shield, which has been off the market for more than 20 years.

Today, two types of IUDs are available: copper IUDs, like the copper T, which remains effective for 5 to 10 years, and progesterone-release IUDs. The latest (approved by the FDA only in

2001) is the Mirena, which slowly releases progesterone and can be left in place as long as five years. The Mirena is being marketed primarily as a treatment for dysfunctional uterine bleeding—or "bleeding for who knows why." It is a very effective method of birth control, with a failure rate of less than 1 percent. The Mirena will probably replace the Progestasert, another progestin-releasing IUD, because the Progestasert must be replaced every year.

IUDs are convenient, but they are probably not the best choice for birth control, at least not in the early postpartum period. In the period after delivery, IUDs can cause infection, bleeding, and scar rupture. For these reasons, we would be very cautious about inserting an IUD in a woman who has recently delivered, and especially a woman who recently had a C-section and has a healing scar. Only you and your doctor can assess your risks versus your potential benefits from the use of an IUD, however.

Injections

Depo-Provera is an injection of medroxyprogesterone acetate, a progestin that is very effective for contraception. Each injection lasts for about three months, at which time another injection is needed. An advantage of Depo-Provera is that it can be used by a breast-feeding mother. Three disadvantages are that it is often associated with weight gain, that it is associated with a risk of osteoporosis, and that it may cause annoying irregular bleeding. The rate of pregnancy for women taking Depo-Provera shots is less than 1 percent.

Lunelle, a combination estrogen-progestin injection that could be administered monthly, was very much like the birth-control pill, except that you only had to think about it once a month. Lunelle is currently unavailable because of concern over the possibility of ineffective dosages.

Implants

Norplant is a device consisting of five rods, each impregnated with slow-release progestin. Norplant is inserted under the skin of the arm through a small incision and is effective for up to five years. A new model, Norplant II, which has just been approved, contains only two rods. Like other progestin-only contraceptives, Norplant and Norplant II can be used immediately after delivery in breast-feeding mothers.

The Future

The NuvaRing, approved by the FDA in early 2002 for use in the United States, sounds like a useful addition to the available hormonally based contraceptives. NuvaRing is an estrogen- and pro-gestin-impregnated ring that you insert in your vagina and leave for three weeks, removing it to allow a withdraw bleed (a period). This device is similar in design to a vaginal ring now available for menopausal women and will probably be just as popular. It is said to have fewer side effects than the pill and, again, just a 1 percent failure rate. It was first available in pharmacies in the summer of 2002.

A new implant, called Implanon, will probably be available in a few years. Implanon is a single rod that slowly releases a steady dose of progestin over a period of three years. It is said to be 100 percent effective and less irritating than the old implant. It is also said to be easier to implant under the skin of the upper arm and then take out three years later. The most common side effects are irritability and other symptoms similar to premenstrual syndrome (PMS).

Another advance in hormonal contraception is Evra, a hormonal patch that can be worn on the upper arm, belly, or buttock, similar to the hormone patch worn by menopausal women. Evra delivers a combination of estrogen and progestin and has a failure rate of about 1 percent. It is worn three weeks out of four, with the fourth week being the week of menstruation. Evra will not come off in the shower or while the woman is swimming. Some women may have difficulty with sensitivity to the adhesive, as with any such product. This product also became available in 2002.

Sterilization

Before even launching on this topic, let us make it clear that female sterilization should be considered a permanent end to childbearing. Please keep that in mind as we discuss female sterilization, especially if you are considering sterilization for yourself.

Any technique for female sterilization involves, in some way, interrupting the Fallopian tubes so sperm can't swim up the tubes to meet the egg. The tubes may be cut, or tied, or cut and tied in this surgery, called *tubal ligation.*

For many people, it makes good sense to have sterilization done while the abdomen is open for another reason—for example, a C-section. Sterilization adds little to the time involved in the surgery, adds nothing to the risks, and avoids the need to have another abdominal procedure. The postop course is not altered at all when a woman has a tubal ligation together with a C-section.

Why would anyone want to be sterilized? Michele and her husband had already decided for a variety of reasons that they would have two children and that their family planning would be easiest if Michele had a tubal ligation with the second C-section. Brenda had her second C-section and a tubal ligation at the same time, and she, too, felt that her family was complete.

Perhaps you have had multiple C-sections and your doctor thinks sterilization would be in your best interest from a medical standpoint. How many Cesarean sections can a woman safely undergo? Obstetricians accept an upper figure of four to five sections but may advise you against another pregnancy at a lower number if your scar seems weak. The risk of rupture of the uterus is considered to increase by 1 percent with each subsequent C-section. Also, adhesions sometimes form between the uterus and surrounding tissue, increasing the risk of rupture and the risk of nicking the bladder each time the abdomen is opened.

Before deciding to be sterilized, anyone, man or woman, should consider all possibilities, including unlikely possibilities such as divorce and remarriage, the death of your spouse, or the death of one of your children. It can be devastating to realize that you really do want another child but can't have one.

Also, be honest with yourself about your emotional readiness for sterilization: some women feel less "womanly" if they do not have the ability to become pregnant. This feeling may have nothing to do with whether they actually *want* another pregnancy, but nevertheless this feeling should not be dismissed. Sterilization is always an option at a later date, if you then feel more comfortable with it. Reversal techniques are widely available today, but they all involve major surgery, they all are very expensive (and often are not covered by insurance), and none of them carries any guarantee of a future pregnancy. What about in vitro fertilization, in which an egg is taken from the ovary, fertilized outside the womb, and then inserted into the womb for gestation? This technology is not available for everyone, it is very expensive (and often not covered by insurance), and the success rate is only 50 percent at best. Be very, very sure that sterilization is what you want.

Many people believe that sterilization is 100 percent effective in preventing pregnancy—but it isn't. And a pregnancy after sterilization doesn't necessarily mean that the procedure wasn't properly done. After ligation, a small number of Fallopian tubes do reconnect on their own, and this occurs slightly more often when the sterilization is done at the time of C-section. Why? The reason has to do with blood supply. The pelvic organs have an excellent blood supply in pregnancy, and the tissues are "plumped out" with high progesterone levels. After these hormone levels drop off, the tissues shrink down. This shrinking, coupled with the good blood supply, can allow the tubes to grow back together. The incidence of pregnancy after sterilization is somewhere between 1 in 200 and 1 in 1,000 women, depending on which procedure is done. (See below for a description of the different approaches to the procedure.)

One other point: pregnancy after sterilization carries a greater than normal risk of tubal pregnancy, though the risk is still small. Tubal pregnancy is a pregnancy developing in the Fallopian tube instead of the uterus. You need to be aware of this risk, however small.

HOW IS IT DONE?

To perform a tubal ligation in conjunction with a C-section, the surgeon has several options. The first choice might be to attach clips to the tubes, similar to putting clothespins on the line. These clips are nonreactive metal and plastic and can stay indefinitely in the abdomen without causing any difficulties. All they do is prevent pregnancy! Of the tubal ligation techniques, this one is the most easily reversed, with a greater than 90 percent success rate when performed by an experienced surgeon.

Another technique involves cutting out a portion of each tube and sewing the cut ends closed. This is like taking a piece out of the middle of a hose and then sewing both exposed ends closed. The success rate in reversing this technique is about 70 percent.

A third technique, which is seldom done today, is total removal of both tubes. This is a difficult technique and very time consuming, so it increases the length of time the patient is anesthetized. This technique may be done during Cesarean section in a woman who became pregnant after a previous, unsuccessful tubal ligation and needed to be delivered by Cesarean.

When tubal ligation is part of Cesarean surgery, the ligation is done after the baby is delivered and the uterus has been sewn back together. Remember, though, that the C-section surgery is not your only opportunity for sterilization. If you later decide that you want to be sterilized, a simple same-day surgery is available. In this surgery, after anesthesia is given, a laparoscope (like a telescope) can be passed through very small (½ to 1 inch) incisions in the abdomen, and the clips can be applied to the tubes through these tiny incisions. This procedure usually involves a few hours' stay in the day-surgery unit of the hospital. Or maybe your partner will opt for a vasectomy. Just be sure about your decision.

MALE STERILIZATION

What *about* male sterilization? This option is called *vasectomy* and involves cutting or clamping the part of the male reproductive organs that deliver sperm from the testes to the urethra.

In each of the two scrotal sacs, there is an almond-shaped organ called the *testis* (commonly called *balls*). Each of the testes is connected to a tube called the *vas deferens*. The vas deferens allows the sperm made in the testis to be transported to the male urethra. The sperm swim down the urethra and then mix with fluids from glands to form the ejaculate that is spurted when the man climaxes.

When a vasectomy is done, the vasa deferentia are cut or clamped to block the passage of the sperm from the testes to the urethra. After a vasectomy, the ejaculate contains no sperm and is therefore sterile.

Vasectomies are often done in a doctor's office or as outpatient surgery in a hospital. The skin of the scrotum is numbed, one or two tiny cuts are made in the skin, and each vas deferens is pulled out into a small loop. The arc of the loop is cut. The raw ends of the severed loop are then stitched, tied, or burned closed to prevent their growing back together. The vas deferens is then slipped back into the scrotum, and the tiny incisions are sutured closed. The whole procedure takes 20 to 30 minutes.

Vasectomy, like tubal ligation, is a permanent method of birth control, and a man must be clear in his own mind that he is at peace with this decision. He must consider the unthinkable "what ifs"—what if he gets a divorce, what if he loses a child? Only after carefully considering these possibilities should anyone consent to sterilization. Vasectomy is minor surgery and has fewer risks and complications than tubal ligation. There is a 0.1 percent chance of unplanned pregnancy after vasectomy.

A point to keep in mind is that the man needs to "clear the system" before relying on his vasectomy as his sole method of contraception. Usually the sperm count is reduced to zero about two months after the vasectomy.

We hope this chapter has provided the information you need to avoid getting pregnant again right away, if you don't want to. Be sure to discuss your contraceptive method with your doctor. Pregnancy and childbirth are such great joys, but it is possible to have too much of a good thing!

CONTRACEPTIVE METHODS

Method	Hor-monal?	Perma-nent?	Convenience
Abstinence	no	no	personal preference
Natural family planning	no	no	personal preference
Condoms	no	no	easily available, cheap
Diaphragm or cervical cap	no	no	Rx; no loss of spontaneity
Sponge	no	no	not currently available
The pill	yes	no	Rx; one pill daily; no loss of spontaneity
Mini-pill	yes	no	same as pill
Copper IUD	no	no	Rx; very convenient
Progesterone IUD	yes	no	same as copper IUD
Depo-Provera	yes	no	Rx; convenient; lasts 3 months
Norplant	yes	no	Rx; effective for 5 years
NuvaRing	yes	no	Rx; worn for 3 weeks
Evra	yes	no	Rx; patch changed weekly
Tubal ligation	no	yes	surgical procedure
Vasectomy	no	yes	minor surgical procedure

Abbreviations: STD, sexually transmitted diseases; Rx, prescription needed.

Failure Rate	Protect against STD?	Health Risks	Comments
none, if strictly adhered to	yes	none	
18–25%, depending on compliance	no	none	
12–18%	yes	none	
12–20%	no	none	Wait 6 wk after C-section
15%	no		
<1%	no	yes	Not while breast-feeding
<1%	no	possible	Not while breast-feeding
<1%	no	yes	Wait 6 wk after C-section
<1%	no	yes	Wait 6 wk after C-section
<1%	no	yes	
<1%	no	yes	
<1%	no	yes	Not while breast-feeding
1%	no	yes	Not while breast-feeding
<0.5%	no	yes	Easy to do at time of C-section
0.2%	no	yes	

CHAPTER 10

ى‍ي   ى‍ي   ى‍ي

Vaginal Birth after Cesarean Section

You remember Jan and Paul from the introduction to this book? When Daniel was one year old, they conceived another child. This was a much more relaxed pregnancy for them. For one thing, they were so busy running after Daniel and dealing with ordinary life, they did not have any time or energy for worrying.

The looming question, however, was whether to try labor or just go for the repeat C-section. Jan felt very conflicted about it, and at 37 weeks, she and Paul visited the obstetrician together to talk about it. After discussing all her concerns, Jan decided that, if she did not go into active labor on her own by her due date, she would have an elective repeat C-section. Making the decision felt like a huge weight off her shoulders.

One week later, very early on a Sunday morning, Jan woke up to heavy pains, already coming five minutes apart. On the way to the hospital, she was pessimistic, thinking: "Here we go again. A poop-out labor and then a section." Much to her surprise and delight, her first exam at the hospital showed that her cervix was already half dilated, at five centimeters. Her doctor came in to examine her and said that she was progressing nicely and that the baby was well into the birth canal. He offered an epidural, knowing how much pain she had had the last time, and she gratefully accepted. Four hours later, a red-faced and squalling Meghan was pushed out by Jan, who was laughing hysterically in her joy.

Jan's vaginal delivery after a previous C-section illustrates a change in thinking in obstetric practice. Until 1981, the dictum always had been that a woman who had one Cesarean section always had to deliver by C-section in the future. (Remember, "once a C-section, always a C-section"?) In 1981, the National Institutes of Health began to encourage a trial of labor after previous C-section. (A *trial of labor* is an attempt to deliver a baby vaginally in circumstances in which there exists a higher-than-normal probability of Cesarean section.) At that time, the rate of vaginal birth after C-section (VBAC) was only 3 percent in the United States; today, 60–80 percent of attempts at trial of labor result in vaginal delivery. (Admittedly, 60–80 percent is a wide spread, but the figures in the medical literature vary this much.)

Currently, there is a movement to decrease the number of surgical births in the United States, including a recommendation for trial of labor for VBAC in some circumstances. This movement is fueled by both philosophical and economic concerns, and it is surrounded by debate (see the introduction). It is neither our interest nor our mandate to participate in this debate in this book. We will make the observation that Healthy People 2000 is a statement of policy objectives (by the U.S. Department of Health and Human Services, joined in 2002 by the National Recreation and Parks Association); Healthy People 2000 advocates a 15 percent C-section rate, which is an apparent average of previous rates and the current rate and is not based on medical studies recommending an optimum rate. Even if we *knew* the optimum rate, each woman's case would have to be assessed individually. Our concern here, therefore, is to provide you with the information you need to make intelligent choices about your own circumstances. In this chapter we look at what goes into a decision to try a trial of labor for vaginal delivery after Cesarean birth.

The American College of Obstetrics and Gynecology has provided clear guidelines for a trial of labor after Cesarean. They state that a trial of labor is appropriate if

- The woman has had one or two lower segment C-sections.
- The woman has a clinically adequate pelvis. (This means that her pelvis is apparently large enough to permit vaginal delivery.)
- There are no scars other than C-section scars on the woman's uterus, and she has not previously had a rupture of the uterus.
- A doctor capable of monitoring the labor and performing an emergency C-section, if necessary, is readily available throughout the labor.
- Anesthesia and personnel are available for emergency C-section.

The guidelines discuss other situations but do not recommend trial of labor other than in the circumstances listed above. An individual woman's chances of success are difficult to predict in advance, but the chances are higher for a woman who has had at least one vaginal delivery.

Diane had delivered two children vaginally, but when she was pregnant with Kyle, he took up his position sprawled across her uterus, crosswise. Nothing would budge him, and he clearly could not be delivered vaginally. So Kyle came by C-section. Two years later, Diane was able to easily and uneventfully deliver Polly vaginally.

Natasha was pregnant with her second child. With her first, Michael, she had had a C-section at 32 weeks because her blood pressure was rising alarmingly. This time, she wanted to do it "on her own." She had no problems with her blood pressure in this pregnancy, and she felt sure that she was going to have a girl. Natasha's labor progressed nicely until her cervix stopped dilating at eight centimeters and just would not go any further. She did not feel cheated when the doctor said it was time for a C-section because she had given labor a good try and had had the experience. Also, she had an epidural in place, ready for a repeat section if needed, and could be awake for the delivery. After Paul was delivered, it was obvious why labor had not progressed: he (not a she!) weighed nine pounds, six ounces. Natasha was delighted with him—and with herself.

Elisabeth had a smiley-face scar from her delivery of twins during an active case of herpes, and she elected to try to deliver her third baby vaginally. She's young and healthy and met all the criteria for a trial of labor. Everything went well in labor until Elisabeth suddenly began to hemorrhage. The staff was standing by, in readiness for emergency C-section, and Elisabeth's baby was promptly delivered by C-section. During the surgery, Elisabeth's doctor discovered that she had a small tear next to her previous scar. This tear probably developed during her labor and was caused by the force of the contractions. All ended well because all of the American College of Obstetrics and Gynecology's criteria were met and C-section was available without delay for Elisabeth.

When a trial of labor is successful, there is no need for a Cesarean section. Because vaginal births result in fewer complications than C-sections, a vaginal birth after C-section is a desirable outcome when possible. As we have noted, however, 20–40 percent of trials of labor are not successful, for any of the reasons for the failure of labor described in this book and for additional reasons resulting from a previous C-section, as happened with Elisabeth. A failed trial of labor results in another emergency C-section. As emergency C-sections result in more complications, such as infections, than either elective repeat C-sections or vaginal deliveries, a trial of labor clearly is not without risk.

The complication most feared by experienced obstetricians is rupture of the uterus—a life-threatening emergency for both the mother and the baby. The risk of rupture during trial of labor with a lower segment, "smiley face" uterine scar is only 0.5–1.5 percent, but it is still a real risk for women who undergo a trial of labor. The scar tissue is very strong, but the wall next to it is relatively weak. Women who have an elective repeat C-section have only a 0.16 percent risk of uterine rupture. A ruptured uterus can make it necessary to perform an emergency hysterectomy to save the mother. A ruptured uterus can also cause damage to the baby. Caroline's patient, Lucy, had uterine rupture during a trial of labor for her second child. The baby died, and Lucy had a hysterectomy in her twenties—truly a tragic ending.

You should *not* have a trial of labor if you have any of the following circumstances:

1. A scar from a prior classical or T-shaped C-section incision or other surgery on the uterus that may weaken it.

2. A contracted pelvis, whether from a birth defect, injury, or illness. A contracted pelvis is a pelvis that is too small to allow vaginal delivery. A previous C-section for failure to progress does not necessarily mean the woman has a contracted pelvis. Labor depends on the strength of contractions and the position of the baby, as well as on the relative "fit" of the baby's head and mother's pelvis.

3. A medical or obstetric complication that precludes vaginal delivery. Linda, for example, now pregnant with her second child, has become diabetic since her daughter, Madison, was delivered by emergency C-section because of an obstructed labor. Women with diabetes often have large babies, so Linda's medical condition makes a repeat C-section a better and safer choice than trial of labor.

4. A situation in which an emergency Cesarean is not immediately available because of lack of facilities or trained personnel. In other words, indulging a trial of labor in a small, rural hospital with no specialist obstetrician or anesthesiologist on staff is flirting with disaster.

A woman who chooses to have a trial of labor may have an epidural, if she wishes, for pain management. The doctor may rupture her membranes to help labor to progress. Intravenous Pitocin or a prostaglandin gel (inserted vaginally) to assist the contractions should be given only with great caution and careful monitoring. Most obstetricians believe that these medications should not be used to induce (start) labor because there is evidence that doing so can increase the risk of uterine rupture.

You should discuss the specifics of your case in detail with your doctor and with your birth partners. Ultimately, this is your choice—unless there are strong medical reasons in favor of or against trial of labor. We have two pieces of advice: keep an open mind about vaginal birth after Cesarean, and remember that a trial of labor is just that—an attempt that may or may not work out.

In your reading, you will probably come across the controversy over rates of C-section and how to decrease the numbers. If you don't, someone who loves you probably will. These concerns have to do with entire populations, not with you as an individual. All that should matter *for you* is to make the decision that is in the best interests of you and your baby, and that decision must be based, as much as possible, on the facts relating to you and your baby. There is no politically or socially *correct* way to have a baby; there is only the best way for you.

APPENDIXES

Questions to Ask Your Doctor

1. Will you be present for the birth of my baby? If not, will you be available if I need a C-section? Who covers for you weekends, holidays, and vacations? Can I meet your backup physician(s) before my due date?

It is common today for doctors who deliver babies to work cooperatively. This only makes good sense, because the safety of the women in their care depends on the doctor not being exhausted from going night after night with little sleep. You need to know who might deliver you if your own physician is not available when you go into labor. In most groups, it is customary for each pregnant woman to see each physician or midwife on at least one of her prenatal visits.

For your safety, your doctor or another doctor who is fully qualified to perform Cesarean sections must either be available on the premises of the hospital or be able to arrive at the hospital within about 20 minutes of receiving a call. This doctor cannot be on call for more than one hospital at the same time—this is imperative.

2. Is an anesthesiologist always present in the hospital, or does an anesthesiologist have to be called in if a C-section is needed?

In major medical centers, there is usually an anesthesiologist present in the hospital; this is simply not possible in rural areas. However, you should be assured that an anesthesiologist is available on call with about 20 minutes arrival time.

3. Should I make an appointment with the anesthesia department before my due date? Does the anesthesia department have any printed material available for patients that describes the types of anesthesia offered in this hospital?

If you are having a planned (elective) C-section, an anesthesia appointment is an expected part of your preparation, but if you are anticipating a vaginal delivery, such an appointment would not be part of your preparation. If you anticipate that you will have an epidural during labor, the procedure should be explained to you before your labor begins. This explanation may come in your prenatal classes, from your doctor or her staff, or through printed materials given to you. Just before this procedure, the anesthesiologist will briefly discuss it with you and give you information specific to you. You will then be asked to sign an informed consent form.

4. Is the room where the C-sections are done in the labor and delivery suite, or is it part of the general surgery suite?

In most hospitals today, the operating room (OR) is a part of the labor and delivery suite. This may not be true in some small, rural hospitals, but the important thing is that the OR be close enough to the delivery room that it would only take about five minutes to transfer you. A woman trying to have a vaginal delivery after a previous C-section should be particularly careful about finding out where the operating room is and how fast she can be transported there if necessary.

5. Can I have my husband or a support person with me in the delivery room? Can this person stay with me if I need to have a C-section?

These days, the answer to this is almost always yes! Discuss this possibility with your husband or support person beforehand. Some people get faint at the thought of being in an OR. It is not selfishness if this person does not want to go into the operating room with you. He or she will be delighted to see you and greet the baby immediately after the birth.

6. What types of monitoring do you do, and what does this hospital do to protect the well-being of my baby? Will my baby's heartbeat be monitored throughout my labor? Will samples of the scalp blood routinely be taken?

Neither continuous monitoring nor routine scalp pH are done in normal labor, nor have these procedures been shown to be necessary or useful. Both of these methods of monitoring the baby should be available for high-risk labor or in the event of problems, however (although neither has been shown to be 100% predictive of a baby's well-being).

7. If I have a C-section, can my baby stay in the same room with me after birth? Can I try breast-feeding right away?

Yes is the preferred answer to both of these questions. Do keep in mind that you may be very tired, especially if you have had a C-section after a long labor, and you may need to sleep first. Usually, hospitals are flexible on these issues.

8. If I am tired and just want to sleep, will the nurses take my baby to the nursery for the night?

We hope so. Both of us remember those as the only good nights of sleep we had for many years! Wee babies tend to wake you up.

9. How soon will I go home? Should I have someone at home to help me?

How soon you go home depends on how well you are healing, peeing, and so on. In most U.S. hospitals today, women are discharged at around day 3. It is certainly a lifesaver to have someone at home to help. In fact, we've devoted a whole chapter of this book to the topic of going home!

Here is one last question, one that is not for your doctor: What if I don't like the answers to these questions?

Be sure you ask these and any other questions you have early in your pregnancy, so you can arrange to go elsewhere for your care, if necessary. It is unusual today for a woman to go along with feeling uncomfortable about her care, and it is not unheard of for a woman to stay with relatives in order to get medical care in a different community. Allow yourself enough time to explore these options.

The Apgar Scale

All babies are scored at one minute and again at five minutes after birth. The Apgar score is a sum of all points assigned for five significant signs: breathing, heart rate, muscle tone, skin color, and reflexes. The highest possible score is a 10, the sum of 2 points in each of the five categories.

The higher the score, the better the baby is doing. The Apgar scale is used to help assess quickly which babies need more specialized resuscitation and attention after birth.

What is tested?	0 point	1 point	2 points
Breathing	absent	slow or irregular	regular
Heart rate	absent	fewer than 100 beats/min	more than 100 beats/min
Muscle tone	limp	some movement	active movements
Skin color	blue	body pink, extremities blue	pink all over
Reflexes	absent	grimace	cry

Calcium-rich Foods

Food	Serving Size	Calcium Content (mg)
Dairy Products		
Milk	8 oz	290
Lactaid plus calcium	8 oz	550
Half & half	4 oz	127
Nonfat dry milk	1 oz	349
Yogurt, plain, low-fat	8 oz	415
Yogurt, plain, whole milk	8 oz	274
Cheese		
American	1 oz	175–190
Cheddar	1 oz	204
Feta	1 oz	140
Monterey Jack	1 oz	211
Mozzarella	1 oz	207
Parmesan	1 oz	355
Ricotta	1 oz	77
Swiss	1 oz	272
Fish		
Anchovies	3 fillets	66
Bass, striped, broiled	4 oz	47
Clams	3 oz	78
Cod, dried, salted	3.5 oz	225
Crab, steamed	3 oz	84
Hake	3.5 oz	41

Herring, canned in brine	3.5 oz	147
Mackerel, canned	1/2 cup	194
Ocean perch	3 oz	117
Oysters, canned	3.5 oz	152
Salmon, broiled, baked	3.5 oz	414
Salmon, red, canned	2/3 cup	259
Sardines, canned in oil/brine	8 sardines	354
Scallops, steamed	3.5 oz	115
Shrimp, raw	3.5 oz	63
Smelt, canned	4–5	358
Trout, brook, cooked	3.5 oz	218
Tuna, albacore, raw	3.5 oz	26

Vegetables

Beans	1 cup	62
Beet greens	1/2 cup	99
Broccoli	2/3 cup	88
Brussels sprouts	6–8	32
Carrots	1 large	37
Chard	1/2 cup	73
Dandelion greens	3.5 oz	187
Kale, raw	3.5 oz	179
Mustard greens, raw	3.5 oz	183
Parsley, raw	3.5 oz	203
Pepper, bell	1 large	9
Pumpkin	1/2 cup	18
Spinach, raw	3.5 oz	93
Sweet potato	1 large	72
Turnip greens, raw	3.5 oz	246
Watercress, raw	3.5 oz	151

Other

Tofu, firm	4 oz	258
Tahini	2 tbsp	128
Almond butter	2 tbsp	44
Brazil nuts	4 nuts	28
Hazelnuts	10–12 nuts	38
Peanut butter	1 tbsp	12
Pecans	12 halves	11
Soynuts	1 oz	68

Iron-rich Foods

Food	Serving Size	Iron Content (mg)
Meat		
Beef	4 oz	3.7
Veal	3.5 oz	3.6
Pork	1 chop	3.9
Lamb	1 chop	2.8
Calf's liver	3.5 oz	14.2
Venison	3.5 oz	3.5
Poultry		
Chicken with skin	3.5 oz	1.25
Turkey	3.5 oz	1.78
Duck	3.5 oz	2.7
Nuts & Seeds		
Almonds	12–15 nuts	0.7
Brazil nuts	4 nuts	0.5
Cashews	6–8 nuts	0.6
Hazelnuts	10–12 nuts	0.5
Peanuts	1 oz	0.85
Soynuts	1 oz	1.4
Walnuts, black	8–10 halves	0.9
Pumpkin seeds	1 oz	3.14
Sesame seeds	1 oz	2.2
Sunflower seeds	1 oz	1.99

Vegetables

Beans	1/2 cup	2.7
Beet greens	3.5 oz	3.3
Broccoli	2/3 cup	0.8
Brussels sprouts	6–8	1.1
Carrots	1 large	0.7
Chard	3.5 oz	3.2
Dandelion greens	3.5 oz	3.1
Kale, raw	3.5 oz	2.2
Mustard greens, raw	3.5 oz	3.0
Parsley, raw	3.5 oz	6.2
Pepper, bell	1 large	0.7
Spinach, raw	3.5 oz	3.1
Spinach, cooked	1/2 cup	2.0
Sweet potato	1 large	1.6
Turnip greens, raw	3.5 oz	1.8
Watercress, raw	3.5 oz	1.7

My Baby Died

In this age of modern technology and health care, death of the baby during delivery or soon after birth is highly unlikely in this country. It does still happen, however, and women who are suffering the grief of losing a child have a special need for emotional support. We want to provide support for anyone who has been touched by the tragedy of infant death.

When we were pregnant, it seemed that everyone wanted to share their worst stories. But a pregnant woman does not need to worry needlessly about something that is so unlikely, and we declined to listen to these stories. The same approach applies to the rest of this chapter: **If you are currently pregnant, do not read the rest of this appendix. Stop here.**

The loss of children, both newborns and older children, used to be a common experience. Thankfully, this situation has changed dramatically in the last 50 years through advances in science, medicine, and technology. Today, the loss of a child is *not* a common experience, but sometimes, even with all our modern advances and knowledge, a child is lost, including, very infrequently, a newborn baby.

When a newborn dies, some unthinking people offer platitudes such as "You're young, you can have more children." These well-intentioned but unhelpful words cannot speak to the grief in your heart. You are grieving, and you must grieve. Grieving is an appropriate response to loss, and the grieving process helps people recover from loss. Know that your partner and your family grieve, too, and honor this. It seems odd to us even to find it necessary to validate the fact that families who have lost a baby need to be permitted to feel their loss in order to be able to heal.

Right after the death of a newborn, nurses on the obstetric floor are very sympathetic and can be helpful. One of the first steps they can take is to help transfer the mother to the surgical floor, where she will not constantly hear babies crying. You may have had this experience. We also hope you encountered a nurse who was sensitive to your needs: some mothers want quiet time—to be given uninterrupted time; others want to talk.

Research shows that an important part of grieving is allowing yourself to know that your baby was a person by, for example, naming him or her. Nurses often will offer to dress the baby in a gown and bonnet and take photos for the family. If you have photographs of your baby, we hope they provide comfort.

Leave-taking rituals have been in place for centuries, and for good reason—they help. You may have turned to your church to conduct such a ritual. A group of your family and friends may have gathered to celebrate this child who has passed through your life and to offer a farewell. Expressing what is in your heart and honoring the individuality of this child whom you knew in utero is part of the grieving process.

Formal support groups include, again, obstetric units whose nurses are trained to help you. Hospice organizations organize and lead grief support groups. Organizations such as Compassionate Friends in the United States are specifically designed to help grieving parents. These organizations understand the stages of grief, including anger, denial, and guilt, and can provide reassurance that all of these feelings are a normal part of grieving and healing.

We encourage any grieving parents to reach out for the support they need; friends and other family members can provide support in many ways and can encourage the parent to make use of available resources to help in grieving. As we said earlier in this chapter, professional grief counselors, psychiatrists, psychologists, social workers, and clergy can provide invaluable assistance in coping with feelings of loss. Please accept our deepest sympathy.

Glossary

Abruptio placentae (ah-**brup**-she-oh pluh-**senn**-tee): a tearing of the placenta from the uterine wall, resulting in bleeding. This bleeding is not normal, and the event is basically an injury to the placenta.

Amniocentesis (**am**-nee-o-senn-**tee**-sis): a diagnostic procedure in which a needle is passed through the mother's abdominal wall into the uterus; through the needle, a small amount of the fluid in which the baby is floating is drawn off into a syringe. This fluid and the cells it contains are then analyzed for the presence of infection, fetal abnormalities, or genetic defects.

Analgesic (an-all-**jee**-sik): a drug that alleviates pain but doesn't produce unconsciousness.

Anemia (ah-**nee**-mee-ah): a condition in which the concentration of red blood cells is lower than normal for the age and sex of the person. Because the red blood cells carry oxygen, anemia decreases the availability of oxygen to the cells of the body.

Anesthetic: a drug that produces insensibility to pain. General anesthetics produce unconsciousness and total insensibility to pain. Regional or local anesthetics produce insensibility or numbing in a particular area of the body and do not affect consciousness.

Antibiotics: substances that are able to destroy or inhibit the growth of bacteria that cause infection.

Anticoagulants (**an**-tee-ko-**ag**-yu-lants): drugs that prevent the blood from clotting. These are important in the treatment of blood clots in the legs or lungs.

Birth canal: the vagina, the muscular passage from the uterus to the exterior.

Birth control: any of a variety of methods used to prevent pregnancy.

Breech presentation: bottom-first positioning of the baby in the uterus.

Catheter (**kath**-uh-ter): a thin, plastic tube inserted in a body part for the purpose of draining or introducing fluids.

Cephalic (seh-**fal**-ik) *presentation:* head-first positioning of the baby in the uterus.

Cephalopelvic (**sef**-ah-low-**pel**-vik) *disproportion:* the baby's head is too large to fit through the mother's birth canal.

Cervix: the lower part, or neck, of the uterus, which protrudes into the vagina.

Cesarean section: a surgical birth, in which the baby is removed from the mother through an incision in the mother's abdomen and uterus. Also called *C-section.*

Cesarean section on demand: a C-section done because the mother wishes to deliver by surgery, not because of medical necessity. Also called *C-section on request.*

Classical incision: a vertical incision in the upper part (or fundus) of the uterus.

Contraception: birth control.

Deep vein thrombosis: blood clot in the deep veins of the legs.

Diabetes: a disease in which the body cannot properly metabolize carbohydrates and sugars. Diabetes in the mother may affect the health of the baby. A woman may develop diabetes for the first time during pregnancy; this is called *gestational diabetes.*

Dilation: the stretching open of the cervix in labor.

Down syndrome: a condition in which the baby has a chromosomal abnormality resulting in a characteristic appearance with an epicanthic fold on the inner part of the eyelid, which gave rise to the old term *mongolism.* Usually the person with Down syndrome has a small nose with a flat bridge and a small mouth. Down syndrome (also called *Down's* syndrome) is usually, though not always, associated with low intelligence. The baby may have heart defects or other health problems.

Dystocia (diss-**toe**-see-ah): when a part of the baby is not able to navigate the birth canal. Shoulder dystocia is not uncommon.

Eclampsia (ek-**lamp**-see-ah): medical condition of pregnancy in which the mother develops high blood pressure, headache, convulsions; eclampsia may lead to coma and death of the mother and baby.

Elective C-section: a Cesarean section performed for medical reasons that are discovered before labor begins. Also called *planned C-section.*

Embolism: a blood clot that develops in the veins of the pelvis or legs and travels through the blood vessels to become lodged in a vital tissue, such as the lungs (pulmonary embolism) or brain (stroke).

Emergency C-section: a Cesarean section performed for unexpected medical reasons that occur during pregnancy or labor. Also called *nonelective C-section.*

Endometriosis (**en**-doe-mee-tree-**oh**-sis): a condition in which endometrial tissue grows abnormally outside the uterus, most commonly on other pelvic structures, such as the Fallopian tubes or ovaries. This condition causes pain, abnormal bleeding, and difficulty in getting pregnant.

Endometrium (en-doe-**mee**-tree-um): the lining of the uterus.

Epidural: regional anesthesia produced by introducing an anesthetic drug through a catheter into the space just outside the membrane covering the spinal cord.

Episiotomy (eh-pees-ee-**ot**-oh-mee): a cut in the tissue between the vaginal opening and the anus, done to help with a vaginal delivery of a baby and/or to prevent a tear of these tissues.

Estrogen: a hormone produced by the ovaries and the placenta. This is the "female" hormone, which is responsible for maintaining breasts and other feminine attributes, normal menstrual cycles, and normal pregnancies.

External version: the attempt to turn a fetus that is in a breech position to the cephalic, or head-first, position by manipulating the baby through the mother's abdomen.

Fallopian tubes: tubes connecting the ovaries and uterus. The sperm swim up the Fallopian tubes to fertilize the egg.

Fetal distress: the condition in which there is a lack of oxygen to the baby's brain and the signs that signal this distress. Fetal distress may be mild, moderate, or severe. Most babies who suffer fetal distress recover completely when delivered in a timely fashion.

Fetal monitoring: electronic tracing of the baby's heart rate, usually done by placing an electrode on the mother's abdomen or in the skin of the baby's scalp.

Fetus: unborn baby in the uterus.

Fibroids (**fie**-broyds): common and benign muscular tumors located in the muscle wall of the uterus. They may be positioned just under the lining of the uterus, in the middle of the muscle wall, or just under the outer covering of the uterus.

Fistula (**fis**-tyou-lah): an opening or tunnel connecting one body cavity with another, for example, between the bladder and the vagina or between the urethra and the vagina.

Folic acid: a B vitamin that is essential in early pregnancy to prevent certain neurological problems in the baby.

Forceps: metal instruments resembling barbecue tongs, which are sometimes used to assist in the vaginal delivery of a baby.

Fundus: the top of the uterus.

Gestation: the length of a pregnancy.

Gestational diabetes: see *diabetes.*

Hemorrhage: bleeding, especially heavy bleeding.

Hormone: a chemical produced by a gland in the body. This chemical travels through the bloodstream to produce a particular effect in another part of the body.

Hypertension: high blood pressure.

Hysterectomy: surgical removal of the uterus.

Incision: a surgical cut.

Incontinence: inability to control the passage of urine or feces.

Intravenous (in-trah-**vee**-nus): directly into a vein and thereby into the bloodstream.

IUD: a device placed inside the uterus to prevent pregnancy (intrauterine device).

Lochia (**low**-key-ah): the bloody discharge after birth.

Lower segment: the lower part of the uterus, located at the top of the cervix.

Lower segment incision: a horizontal incision in the lower part of the uterus, just at the top of the cervix.

Meconium (mee-**ko**-nee-um): the bowel contents of the fetus. Meconium passed into the birth waters is a sign of fetal distress. Ordinarily, meconium is passed as the baby's feces over the first few days after birth.

Membranes: the protective coverings surrounding the baby in the uterus. The membranes also enclose the fluid that cushions the baby against trauma in the womb.

Morbidity: damage or disease.

Mortality: death.

Neurological: having to do with the nervous system.

Nonelective C-section: a Cesarean section performed for unexpected medical reasons that occur during pregnancy or labor. Also called *emergency C-section.*

Ovary: one of two almond-shaped organs located on either side of the uterus. The ovaries produce hormones and store and release eggs.

Ovum: egg.

Oxytocin (ok-see-**toe**-sin): a hormone produced by the pituitary gland, which is located in the brain. Oxytocin stimulates the uterus to contract and the breasts to produce milk.

Paralytic ileus (**ill**-ee-us): a condition in which the muscles of the gut cannot produce the rhythmic movements that expel feces; can be associated with the trauma of abdominal surgery.

Pelvic floor: the girdle of muscle located inside the pelvis which supports the pelvic organs, such as the uterus and bladder.

Pelvis: the bony cage to which the hips are attached.

Perineum (**pear**-ih-**nee**-um): the area of flesh between the vagina and anus.

Peritoneum (**pear**-ih-toe-**nee**-um): the clear membrane covering the uterus, tubes, bowel, and all internal organs.

Peritonitis (**pear**-ih-toe-**nigh**-tis): inflammation of the peritoneum.

Pfannenstiel incision: the "bikini" or smiley-face incision.

Pitocin: synthetic oxytocin.

Placenta: the blood-rich tissue that develops on the inner wall of the uterus during pregnancy. The placenta is connected to the fetus through the umbilical cord and provides the fetus with oxygen and nutrients.

Placenta previa: a condition in which the placenta is located, either partially or completely, low in the uterus, near or over the birth canal, such that it may tear when labor begins.

Placental insufficiency: inability of the placenta to provide adequate nutrients and oxygen to the fetus.

Planned C-section: a Cesarean section performed for medical reasons that are discovered before labor begins. Also called *elective C-section.*

Pre-eclampsia (pree-ee-**klamp**-sea-ah): a condition in pregnancy in which the mother's blood pressure rises, she spills protein into her urine, and she becomes bloated with retained fluid.

Presentation: the part of the fetus lying nearest the cervix and vagina.

Progesterone: a hormone produced by the ovaries and placenta.

Progestin (pro-**jes**-tin): synthetic progesterone.

Prolapse: the descent into the vagina of the uterus or vaginal walls, also affecting the urethra, bladder, and/or rectum.

Prolapsed cord: a condition during labor or delivery in which the umbilical cord falls into the vagina, where it can be compressed, cutting off oxygen from the baby.

Ruptured membranes: a tear in the membranes so that the waters drain out, which may occur spontaneously or because the doctor or midwife breaks the membranes for a medical reason.

Shoulder dystocia (diss-**toe**-see-ah): difficulty in delivering the shoulders of the baby after the head has been successfully delivered in a vaginal delivery.

Spinal anesthesia: regional anesthesia produced by introducing an anesthetic through a needle into the fluid surrounding the spinal cord.

Thrombosis: a blood clot forming in the veins, usually in the legs or pelvis.

Toxemia: old term for *pre-eclampsia.*

Transverse lie: the fetus lying directly across the uterus, horizontally.

Trial of labor: an attempt to deliver a baby vaginally in circumstances with a probability of Cesarean section. Often used for an attempt to deliver vaginally after a previous C-section.

Ultrasound: obtaining an image of an internal organ or the fetus by using sound waves.

Urethra: the tube from the bladder to the exterior of the body, which allows the passage of urine.

Uterus: the hollow muscular organ that sits in the pelvis between the bladder and the rectum. The fetus develops in the uterus.

Vagina: the muscular passage from the uterus to the exterior of the body.

Water: the fluid around the baby in the uterus, surrounded by membranes.

Womb: uterus.

Resources

Books on Childbirth and Cesarean Delivery

C. Costanzo et al. *The Twelve Gifts of Birth*. New York: Harper Collins, 2001.

K. Crawford et al. *Natural Childbirth after Cesarean: A Practical Guide*. Malden, Mass.: Blackwell Science, 1996.

S. Datta. *Childbirth and Pain Relief: An Anesthesiologist Explains Your Options*. Chester, N.J.: Next Decade, 2001.

A. Douglas and J. R. Sussman. *The Unofficial Guide to Having a Baby*. New York: Hungry Minds, 1999.

A. C. Harris. *The Pregnancy Journal: A Day-to-Day Guide to a Happy and Healthy Pregnancy*. San Francisco: Chronicle Books, 1996.

R. V. Johnson, ed. *Mayo Clinic Complete Book of Pregnancy and Baby's First Year*. New York: William Morrow, 1994.

E. Kaufmann. *Vaginal Birth after Cesarean: The Smart Woman's Guide to VBAC*. Alameda, Calif.: Hunter House, 1996.

D. Korte. *The VBAC Companion: The Expectant Mother's Guide to Vaginal Birth after Cesarean*. Boston: Harvard Common Press, 1998.

B. Luke and T. Eberlein. *When You're Expecting Twins, Triplets, or Quads: A Complete Resource*. New York: Harper Perennial Library, 1999.

L. Nilsson. *A Child Is Born*. New York: Delacorte Press/Seymour Lawrence, 1990.

L. B. Richards, ed. *The Vaginal Birth after Cesarean Experience: Birth Stories by Parents and Professionals*. Westport, Conn.: Bergin & Garvey, 1990.

W. Sears and M. Sears. *The Birth Book: Everything You Need to Know to Have a Safe and Satisfying Birth*. Boston: Little, Brown, 1994.

W. Sears et al. *The Pregnancy Book: Month-by-Month, Everything You Need to Know from America's Baby Experts.* Boston: Little, Brown, 1997.

Books about Breast-feeding

M. S. Eiger and S. W. Olds. *The Complete Book of Breastfeeding.* New York: Bantam Books, 1999.

C. Martin et al. *The Nursing Mother's Problem Solver.* New York: Simon & Schuster, 2000.

G. Pryor. *Nursing Mother, Working Mother: The Essential Guide for Breastfeeding and Staying Close to Your Baby after You Return to Work.* Boston: Harvard Common Press, 1997.

M. Renfrew et al. *Breastfeeding: Getting Breastfeeding Right for You.* Berkeley, Calif.: Celestial Arts, 2000.

W. Sears and M. Sears. *The Breastfeeding Book: Everything You Need to Know about Nursing Your Child from Birth through Weaning.* Boston: Little, Brown, 2000.

J. Tamaro. *So That's What They're For! Breastfeeding Basics.* Holbrook, Mass.: Adams Media, 1998.

Books about Postpartum Depression

C. Aiken. *Surviving the Post-natal Depression: At Home, No One Hears You Scream.* London: Jessica Kingley Publishers, 2000.

A. M. Huysman. *A Mother's Tears: Understanding the Mood Swings that Follow Childbirth.* New York: Seven Stories Press, 1998.

L. Madsen. *Rebounding from Childbirth.* New York: Bergin & Garvey, 1994.

M. Osmond et al. *Behind the Smile: My Journey out of Postpartum Depression.* New York: Warner Books, 2001.

S. Placksin. *Mothering the New Mother: Women's Feelings and Needs after Childbirth. A Support and Resource Guide.* New York: Newmarket Press, 2000.

Fiction

R. Dorrestein. *A Heart of Stone.* New York: Viking Books, 2001.

Helpful Websites

www.obgyn.net/femalepatient/default.asp?page=leopold
www.alexian.org/progserv/babies/birthto3m/severe.html
pregnancytoday.com/reference/articles/seafood.htm
dacc.uchicago.edu/manuals/obstetric/obanesthesia.html

Postpartum Support International:
  www.chss.iup.edu/postpartum/postpart.html
  postpartum@aol.com
  jhonikman@earthlink.net
  kruckman@grove.iup.edu

Selected Bibliography

Ali Y. Analysis of cesarean delivery in Jimma Hospital, south-western Ethiopia. *East African Medical Journal* 72 (January 1995): 60–63.

Al-Mufti R, McCarthy A, Fisk N. Survey of obstetricians' personal preference and discretionary practice. *European Journal of Obstetrics, Gynecology, and Reproductive Biology* 73 (1997): 1–4.

Atkinson SJ, Farias MF. Perceptions of risk during pregnancy amongst urban women in northeast Brazil. *Social Science and Medicine* 41 (1995): 1577–86.

Boerma JT. The magnitude of the maternal mortality problem in sub-Saharan Africa. *Social Science and Medicine* 24 (1997): 551–59.

Boyce PM, Todd AL. Increased risk of postnatal depression after emergency caesarean section. *Medical Journal of Australia* 157 (August 1992): 172–74.

Cai W-W, Marks JS, Chen CHC, Zhuang Y-X, Morris L, Harris JR. Increased cesarean section rates and emerging patterns of health insurance in Shanghai, China. *American Journal of Public Health* 88 (1998): 777–80.

Danso KA, Martey JO, Wall LL, Elkins TE. The epidemiology of genitourinary fistulae in Kumasi, Ghana, 1977–1992. *International Urogynecologic Journal of Pelvic Floor Dysfunction* 7, no. 3 (1996): 117–20.

de Mello e Souza C. C-sections as ideal births: the cultural constructions of beneficence and patients' rights in Brazil. *Cambridge Questions of Health Ethics* 3 (Summer 1994): 358–66.

Doh AS. A clinical study of cesarean section at the University Teaching Hospital (C.H.U.) Yaounde (1982–1989). *Central African Journal of Medicine* 37 (October 1991): 326–28.

Elhag BI, Milaat WA, Taylouni ER. An audit of cesarean section among Saudi females in Jeddah, Saudi Arabia. *Journal of the Egyptian Public Health Association* 79, no. 1 (1994): 2.

Erkaya S, Tuncer RA, Kutlar I, Onat N, Ercakmak S. Outcome of 1040 consecutive breech deliveries: clinical experience of a maternity hospital in Turkey. *International Journal of Gynaecology and Obstetrics* 59 (November 1997): 115–18.

Faure EAM. Anesthesia for the Pregnant Patient. Department of Anesthesia and Critical Care, University of Chicago, May 2000. http://dacc.uchicago.edu/manuals/obstetric/obanesthesia.html.

Gamble A. Is Seafood Safe during Pregnancy? *Pregnancy Today* http://pregnancytoday.com/reference/articles/seafood.htm.

Garite TJ, Dildy GA, McNamara H, Nageotte MP, Boehm FH, Dellinger EH, Knuppel RA, Porreco RP, Miller HS, Sunderji S, Varner MW, Swedlow DB. A multicenter controlled trial of fetal pulse oximetry in the intrapartum management of nonreassuring fetal heart rate patterns. *American Journal of Obstetrics and Gynecology* 183 (November 2000): 1049–58.

Geary M, Wilshin J, Persaud M, Hindmarsh PC, Rodeck CH. Do doctors have an increased rate of Cesarean section? *Lancet* 18 (April 1998): 351.

Glazener CM, Abdalla M, Stroud P, Naji S, Templeton A, Russell IT. Postnatal maternal morbidity: extent, causes, prevention and treatment. *British Journal of Obstetrics and Gynaecology* 102 (1995): 282–87.

Gomes UA, Silva AA, Bettiol H, Barbieri MA. Risk factors for the increasing caesarean section rate in Southeast Brazil: a comparison of two birth cohorts, 1978–1979 and 1994. *International Journal of Epidemiology* 28 (August 1999): 687–94.

Gomez OL, Carrasquilla G. Factors associated with unjustified Cesarean section in four hospitals in Cali, Colombia. *International Journal of Quality in Health Care* 11, no. 5 (1999): 385–89.

Hannah ME, et al. Outcomes at three months after planned Cesarean *vs* planned vaginal delivery for breech presentation at term: the International Randomized Term Breech Trial. *Journal of the American Medical Association* 287 (April 2000): 1822.

Hilton P, Ward A. Epidemiological and surgical aspects of urogenital fistulae: a review of 25 years experience in southeast Nigeria. *International Urogynecologic Journal of Pelvic Floor Dysfunction* 9, no. 4 (1998): 189–94.

Hudson CN. Elective caesarean section for prevention of vertical transmission of HIV-1 infection. *Lancet* 27 (March 1999): 353.

Inter-Agency Group for Safe Motherhood. The safe motherhood action agenda: priorities for the next decade. Report on the Safe Motherhood Technical Consultation, 18–23 October 1997, Colombo, Sri Lanka.

Konje JC, Obisesan KA, Ladipo OA. Obstructed labor in Ibadan. *International Journal of Gynaecology and Obstetrics* 39 (September 1992): 17–21.

Lam SK. Caesarean on request. *Lancet* 20 (March 1993): 341.

Lennox CE, Kwast BE, Farley TM. Breech labor on the WHO partograph. *International Journal of Gynaecology and Obstetrics* 62 (August 1998): 117–27.

Lydon-Rochelle M, Holt VL, Easterling TR, Martin DP. Risk of uterine rupture during labor among women with a prior Cesarean delivery. *New England Journal of Medicine* 345 (5 July 2001): 3–8.

Mahler H. The Safe Motherhood Initiative: a call to action. *Lancet* 1 (1987): 668–70.

Mould TAJ, Chong S, Spencer JAD, Gallivan S. Women's involvement with the decision preceding their caesarean section and their degree of satisfaction. *British Journal of Obstetrics and Gynaecology* 103 (November 1996): 1074–77.

Murray SF, Serani Pradenas F. Cesarean birth trends in Chile, 1986 to 1994. *Birth* 24 (December 1997): 258–63.

Notzon FC. International differences in the use of obstetric interventions. *Journal of the American Medical Association* 263 (27 June 1990): 3286–91.

Nuttall C. Caesarean section controversy: the caesarean culture of Brazil. *British Medical Journal* 320 (15 April 2000): 1074.

Pai M, Sundaram P, Radhakrishnan KK, Thomas K, Muliyil JP. A high rate of caesarean sections in an affluent section of Chennai: is it cause for concern? *National Medical Journal of India* 12 (July–August 1999): 156–58.

Parada OH, Winograd RH, Tomassini TL. Cesarean birth epidemics. *American Journal of Obstetrics and Gynecology* 177 (5 July 1997): 249.

Rice PL, Naksook C. Caesarean or vaginal birth: perceptions and experience of Thai women in Australian hospitals. *Australian and New Zealand Journal of Public Health* 22 (August 1998): 604–8.

Roberts H. Washington diarist: push and pull. *New Republic,* 19 November 2001, p. 50.

Schnapp C, Sepulveda W. Rise in caesarean births in Chile. *Lancet* 349 (4 January 1997): 64.

Starrs A. *Preventing the Tragedy of Maternal Deaths: A Report on the International Safe Motherhood Conference, Nairobi, February 1987,* 56. Geneva: World Bank, 1987.

Stephenson PA, Bakoula C, Hemminki E, Knudsen L, Levasseur M, Schenker J, Stembera Z, Tiba J, Verbrugge HP, Zupan J, Wagner MG, Karagas M, Pizacani B, Pineault R, Tuimala R, Houd S, Lomas J. Patterns of use of obstetrical interventions in 12 countries. *Paediatric and Perinatal Epidemiology* 7 (1993): 45–54.

Sultan AH, Stanton SL. Preserving the pelvic floor and perineum during childbirth—elective caesarean section? *British Journal of Obstetrics and Gynaecology* 103 (1996): 731–34.

Tadesse E, Adane M, Abiyou M. Caesarean section deliveries at Tikur Anbessa Teaching Hospital, Ethiopia. *East African Medical Journal* 73 (September 1996): 629–32.

Task Force on Obstetrical Anesthesia. Practice Guidelines for Obstetrical Anesthesia. American Society of Anesthesiologists, 1999. www.asahq.org/practice/ob/obguide.html.

Tatar M, Gunalp S, Somunoglu S, Demirol A. Women's perceptions of cesarean section: reflections from a Turkish teaching hospital. *Social Science and Medicine* 50 (May 2000): 1227–33.

van Enk A, Doornbos HPR, Nordbeck HJ. Some characteristics of labor in ethnic minorities in Amsterdam. *International Journal of Gynaecology and Obstetrics* 33 (1990): 307–11.

Walraven G, Scherf C, West B, Ekpo G, Paine K, Coleman R, Bailey R, Morison L. The burden of reproductive-organ disease in rural women in The Gambia, West Africa. *Lancet* 14 (April 2001); 357: 1161–67.

Weil O, Fernandez H. Is safe motherhood an orphan initiative? *Lancet* 11 (September 1999); 354: 940–43.

Wirakusumah FF. Maternal and perinatal mortality/morbidity associated with cesarean section in Indonesia. *British Journal of Obstetrics and Gynaecology* 21 (October 1995): 475–81.

Ziadeh SM, Sunna EI. Decreased cesarean birth rates and improved perinatal outcome: a seven-year study. *Birth* 22 (September 1995): 144–47.

Index